T0271110

Animal Ethics in Animal Research

The use of animals in research has always been surrounded by ethical controversy. This book provides an overview of the central ethical issues focussing on the interconnectedness of science, law and ethics. It aims to make theoretical ethical reasoning understandable to non-ethicists and provide tools to improve ethical decision-making on animal research. It focuses on good scientific practice, the 3Rs (replacement, reduction and refinement), ethical theories applied to specific cases and an overview of regulatory issues. The book is co-authored by experts in animal research, animal welfare, social sciences, law and ethics, and provides both animal researchers and members of animal ethics committees with knowledge that can facilitate their work and communication with stakeholders and the public. The book is written to provide knowledge, not to argue a certain position, and is intended to be used in training that aims to fulfil EU Directive 2010/63/EU.

Helena Röcklinsberg is Associate Professor in Ethics at the Swedish University of Agricultural Sciences, teaching ethics in animal science and veterinary education, as well as performing research on ethical issues in relation to animals and food in interdisciplinary research groups.

Mickey Gjerris is Associate Professor in the Department of Food and Resource Economics at the University of Copenhagen, researching and teaching animal ethics, environmental ethics, bioethics, medical ethics and climate ethics.

I. Anna S. Olsson is a researcher and research group leader in laboratory animal welfare and animal research ethics. She coordinates training for researchers using animals and is engaged in ethics review and policy-making for animal-based research at the institutional as well as the European level.

Animal Ethics in Animal Research

HELENA RÖCKLINSBERG
Swedish University of Agricultural Sciences

MICKEY GJERRIS
University of Copenhagen

I. ANNA S. OLSSON
IBMC/i3S, University of Porto

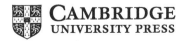

CAMBRIDGE
UNIVERSITY PRESS

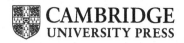
CAMBRIDGE
UNIVERSITY PRESS

Shaftesbury Road, Cambridge CB2 8EA, United Kingdom

One Liberty Plaza, 20th Floor, New York, NY 10006, USA

477 Williamstown Road, Port Melbourne, VIC 3207, Australia

314–321, 3rd Floor, Plot 3, Splendor Forum, Jasola District Centre, New Delhi – 110025, India

103 Penang Road, #05–06/07, Visioncrest Commercial, Singapore 238467

Cambridge University Press is part of Cambridge University Press & Assessment, a department of the University of Cambridge.

We share the University's mission to contribute to society through the pursuit of education, learning and research at the highest international levels of excellence.

www.cambridge.org
Information on this title: www.cambridge.org/9781108420617

DOI: 10.1017/9781108354882

First published 2017

A catalogue record for this publication is available from the British Library

Library of Congress Cataloging-in-Publication data
Names: Röcklinsberg, Helena, author. | Gjerris, Mickey, author. |
S. Olsson, I. Anna, author.
Title: Animal ethics in animal research / Helena Röcklinsberg,
Mickey Gjerris, I. Anna S. Olsson.
Description: Cambridge, United Kingdom; New York, NY: Cambridge
University Press, 2017. | Includes bibliographical references and index.
Identifiers: LCCN 2017025036 | ISBN 9781108420617 (hardback) |
ISBN 9781108430685 (paperback)
Subjects: | MESH: Animal Experimentation – ethics |
Ethics, Research | Animal Welfare
Classification: LCC HV4708 | NLM W 20.55.A5 | DDC 179/.3–dc23
LC record available at https://lccn.loc.gov/2017025036

ISBN   978-1-108-42061-7   Hardback
ISBN   978-1-108-43068-5   Paperback

Contents

Notes on the Authors

There are three main authors of this book. Helena Röcklinsberg, who initiated and was the coordinator of the project, is an animal ethicist at the Swedish University of Agricultural Sciences, Uppsala, sharing her time between teaching and supervising at all animal science programs, from bachelor level to doctoral students, and performing research in animal ethics and food ethics. She is also a member of the committee for ethics and education in animal research at the Swedish Board of Agriculture since its establishment in 2008. Mickey Gjerris is a bioethicist at The University of Copenhagen where he for more than 15 years has been doing research in (among other subjects) animal ethics and has taught courses for veterinarians, researchers and animal caretakers both at the university and for private companies. I. Anna S. Olsson is an animal welfare scientist at the University of Porto, Institute for Research and Innovation in Health, where she is developing research into the behaviour and welfare of laboratory animals and ethical aspects of animal use, organizes training in laboratory animal science for researchers and technicians, and coordinates the animal ethics committee.

Preface

Most people will agree that it is wrong to subject another sentient being to pain, distress, frustration, mental suffering and death. However, most will also agree that there are exceptions to this very general rule. The first one is that we sometimes have to subject someone to suffering to help them – even though we cannot explain this to them. That is typically the situation when we take our family animals and even our small children to the clinic to get them vaccinated. Yet, as it is something that is done to benefit the animal or child in question, very few would find this wrong. The other exception is when the expected end results seem to justify us doing it. Modern warfare notoriously creates 'collateral damage' – civilians hurt or killed by the conflict even though they have nothing to do with it. The justification does not remove the sadness and the tragedy, but many will still find it justified to – under certain conditions – enter into armed conflict to protect democratic societies.

The world of research animals falls into this second category of exceptions. We use animals in a multitude of ways to create new knowledge, check the validity of existing knowledge, train doctors and veterinarians in surgical procedures, test medical compounds for human safety and so on. None of this is done with malicious intent, but to achieve what many find are laudable goals. This does not mean, however, that there are no ethical issues involved in using animals in research. The most obvious question is when it is justified to use animals for purposes that are not in their own best interest. But questions evoked within the research process also arise, e.g. how to handle and house the animals, which animals to use, how to implement the 3Rs into research practice, what minimum level of welfare the animals are entitled to and whether the death of the animal, irrespective of the way it comes about, carries ethical significance. Further, genetic modification of animals into e.g. disease models models raise a number of ethical issues.

A wide range of ethical issues have long been recognized in the research world, among those taking care of the animals, among ethicists and other scholars studying the relationship between humans and animals, and in public discussions. In this book we focus on the core ethical considerations evoked by everyday animal research and present and discuss central ethical theories and a number of relevant concepts such as animal welfare, rights and integrity.

The purpose of this book is not to say who is right and who is wrong. We do not pretend to hold the answers, but we do hope to inspire qualified discussions and help people working in the world of research animals to better grasp and elaborate on the issues. We are, so to speak, not looking to tell our readers what they should think, but to help them make informed decisions and qualify their opinions on these matters.

The book focuses on the ethical, legal and social issues related to the use of animals in research and is aimed at readers who have no or only little prior theoretical experience with these issues. The book presents a range of issues with relevance for animal research such as research design, the 3Rs, animal welfare, public perceptions, public participation, animal ethics, legislative frameworks etc., and introduces the reader to the ethical and philosophical background of these areas. As such, it is an introduction to the range of philosophical reasoning possible in relation to the use of animals in research, not a comprehensive presentation of these theories. We consider this approach important for professionals in animal research, as the new regulation within the European Union Directive (2010/63/EU) requires not only mandatory training to obtain permission to work with research animals but also that this training include ethics. We envisage this textbook to be used as the basic curriculum at such training courses, as it covers ethical considerations, practical considerations and an overview of the legal framework in which the use of animals in research is embedded.

The book aims at considering and discussing issues relevant to professionals holding different roles, e.g. technicians, students, researchers, veterinarians as well as teachers, members of animal ethics committees and policy makers. We focus on an EU context and give an elaborate description of the North American situation in order to cover the regions known to perform most of the world's animal-based research governed by detailed legislation and established guidelines and assessment structures. With few exceptions, the issues and perspectives presented are internationally relevant, and hence we hope that the book will be useful to researchers in other parts of the world as well.

Against this background, the book has a clear goal: to help the reader see the values embedded in the discussions and the complexity and interrelatedness of the many issues in using animals for research purposes. We also intend to show the context of ethical discussions concerning research animals. When working with research animals, it is important to understand not only the ethical issues but also the practical context. How are the animals used and for what purposes? What does it mean to implement the 3Rs? What are the legal requirements both in the EU and in other countries with which one might collaborate? What methods exist to involve a broader public, and what are good reasons for doing so? As a whole, the book gives a complete coverage of animal research ethics. The chapters have been written so that they can be used as stand-alone texts, in order to better serve a wide readership with different background knowledge, but we believe that a comprehensive understanding of the field can best be achieved by reading the whole book. Our main hope is that this will encourage and enable animal researchers and animal technicians to enter ethical discussions and to facilitate such.

The book consists of seven chapters that cover different aspects of the practical, ethical and legal issues connected to research animals. Chapter 1 describes issues related to research ethics in general and to designing animal research especially, elaborating on the interconnectedness of research ethics, animal ethics, animal welfare and research design; it also considers ethical deliberations in animal ethics committees. In Chapter 2 we present the most used and known normative ethical theories and discuss their stance on the use of animals in research. Chapter 3 contains a discussion of what 'good scientific practice' means when applied to the area of research animals, focusing on the concept of animal welfare, how it can be applied, the classification of degree of severity as well as a discussion of how to interpret the 3Rs. The first three chapters are closely linked to Chapter 4 in which six recent examples of animal-based research are presented and scrutinized from the position of the ethical theories. The chapter concludes with a discussion of the role of social aspects for evaluation of research. Chapter 5 differs somewhat from other chapters not only in terms of its length but also because it holds less of discussion; instead, it presents an overview of relevant legislation in many parts of the world. The main focus is on the EU and the recent directive on research animals, as well as the legislation and ethical assessment process in North America, but the chapter also includes descriptions of the regulations in Asia, Australia and Latin America, followed by a presentation of a number of guidelines developed by the research community itself.

As legislation is at least in part meant to meet public concerns about animal research, we focus on public involvement in Chapter 6. Although there is often public concern about the use of animals in research, the possibilities for the public to get involved differ. The chapter ends with a discussion of how public involvement can take place, as public involvement is crucial for public support. Finally, in Chapter 7 we elaborate on alternatives to use of animals, and try to look into the crystal ball and provide a guesstimate on where both the use of research animals and the ethical discussions connected to it can go in the future.

Please note that after each chapter there are a few questions that can be used to discuss the main points of the chapter. There are also references after each chapter that can be used as a resource for further information, and an index of key terms and authors at the end of the book.

Acknowledgements

The three main authors have included a series of co-authors, each experts within their fields, to ensure that the knowledge presented here is comprehensive and correct. At the beginning of each chapter (or section) the readers will be able to see who has contributed and what their affiliation is. We would like to thank all co-authors for sharing their knowledge and time. As already mentioned, the world of research animals is complex, spanning scientific categories from veterinary medicine, biomedical science and law to social sciences and philosophy. This book would not have been possible without contributions from the co-authors representing these and other fields.

Besides the contributors, a range of people have helped make this book a reality. They have read the book and provided helpful and constructive criticism, helped us identify relevant pictures and sources of information, and provided other valuable assistance. A special thanks goes out to:

Klas Abelson, PhD, Associate Professor, Faculty of Health and Medical Sciences, University of Copenhagen, Denmark

Dorte Bratbo Sørensen, DVM, PhD, Associate Professor, Faculty of Health and Medical Sciences, University of Copenhagen, Denmark

Peter Bollen, PhD, Head of section, Faculty of Health and Medical Sciences, University of Southern Denmark, Denmark

Gilly Griffin, PhD, Director of Standards, Canadian Council of Animal Care, Ottawa, Canada

María José Höztel, Professor in Animal Science, Federal University of Santa Catarina, Brazil

Rikke Langebæk, PhD, DVM, Senior veterinarian Faculty of Health, University of Copenhagen, Denmark

Anders Nordgren, Professor of Bioethics, Linköping University, Sweden

Karin Sandstedt, PhD, DVM, researcher, Karolinska Institutet, Stockholm, Sweden

Orsolya E. Varga, PhD, researcher, Faculty of Public Health, University of Debrecen, Hungary

Alexandra Whittaker, LLB VetMB PhD, The University of Adelaide, Australia

We are grateful to our editors at Cambridge University Press for most insightfull support, and to João Duarte and to Claes Anderson, who helped with the final editing. Finally we owe a special thank to Elisabeth Tjärnström, who efficiently assisted us with literature search, editing the manuscript and improving the structure of chapters and content.

All these individuals have helped improve the book; all remaining errors, mistakes and shortcomings are those of the three main authors. Last but not least, we are grateful to our families for support and understanding during the process. Without them we would not have had energy and courage to make this book.

WITH CONTRIBUTIONS BY

Katarina Cvek, PhD, Coordinator of animal research, Faculty of Veterinary Medicine and Animal Sciences, Swedish University of Agricultural Sciences, Uppsala, Sweden

Joana Fernandes, MSc, Research assistant, IBMC – Instituto de Biologia Molecular e Celular, i3S - Instituto de Investigação e Inovação em Saúde, Universidade do Porto, Porto, Portugal

Franz Gruber, DVM, Assoc. Prof., President Doerenkamp-Zbinden Foundation and CEO ALTEX Edition, Kuesnacht, Switzerland

Javier Guillén, DVM, Senior Director for Europe and Latin America, AAALAC International, Pamplona, Spain

Jesper Lassen, PhD, Professor in the sociology of food and agriculture, Faculty of Science, University of Copenhagen, Denmark

Thomas Bøker Lund, PhD, Associate Professor, Faculty of Science, University of Copenhagen, Denmark

Franck L.B. Meijboom, Associate Professor in Ethics, Ethics Institute, Utrecht University, the Netherlands

Karin Gabrielsson Morton, Senior policy advisor, Swedish Fund for Research Without Animal Experiments, Stockholm, Sweden

Elisabeth Ormandy, PhD, Executive Director, Animals in Science Policy Institute, Vancouver, Canada

Jan Lund Ottesen, DVM, PhD, dipECLAM, Vice President Laboratory Animal Science, Maaloev, Novo Nordisk

Catherine Schuppli, PhD, DVM, Clinical Veterinarian, Animal Care Services and Clinical Assistant Professor, Faculty of Land and Food Systems, University of British Columbia, Vancouver, Canada

Mats Sjöquist, Professor, Director of Swedish Center for Animal Welfare, Swedish University of Agricultural Sciences, Uppsala, Sweden

Orsolya E. Varga, PhD, researcher, Faculty of Public Health, University of Debrecen, Hungary

Catarina Vieira de Castro, PhD, postdoctoral research fellow, IBMC – Instituto de Biologia Molecular e Celular, i3S – Instituto de Investigação e Inovação em Saúde, Universidade do Porto, Porto, Portugal

I   Research Ethics

Many countries have legislation regulating research on humans and animals, as well as on how to handle information from humans participating in a study. In addition, there are guidelines for universities, industry and funding bodies (see Chapter 5). Legislation and guidelines are, however, not always enough to ensure a good scientific practice, as even the clearest guidelines and laws need to be interpreted by those working within their framework. The individual researcher or research group still has to discuss and decide how to implement the ethical values underlying legislation and guidelines in their everyday work. In this chapter we outline the most important discussions within the area of research ethics as they relate to core issues in animal-based research.

I.I   CHALLENGES IN THE RESEARCH PROCESS: THE NEED FOR RESEARCH INTEGRITY

Research integrity (also known as responsible conduct of research) is relevant to research performed in all scientific disciplines, as its focus is on ethical issues evoked in and by research as such. Hence, depending on the discipline, somewhat different issues are at stake. For example, in anthropology, medicine, psychology and sociology, issues related to involving or using informants are frequent, whereas research ethical issues in history or geography rather concern how to use documents and research material in a correct way; across all disciplines, research making statistical analyses needs to be concerned with relevance, reliability and validity. Independent of disciplines, a number of areas and issues are relevant to consider in order to ensure good research practice: research planning and conduct; data management; publication and communication; authorship management;

collaboration practices; and conflicts of interest (see e.g. Danish Code of Conduct for Research Integrity [Ministry of Higher Education and Science, 2014]).

Scientific misconduct and questionable conduct of research can occur within in all these spheres. Examples of misconduct are fabrication of data (creating data 'out of thin air'), falsification of data (inclusion or exclusion of data to falsely underpin a certain result) and plagiarism (using own or someone else's text or material without accurate reference). Examples of questionable conduct of research are accepting or granting undeserved authorships, using inappropriate methodologies and failing to acknowledge contributions from others. Due to time and resource limits, verification of research, i.e. repetition, might not always be done, whereby false results are spread. Further, dishonesty in relation to funding bodies and publishing the same study in several contexts reveal lack of professionalism and poor research ethics (ESF, 2011).

There are many reasons for researchers to adhere to responsible conduct of science. For one thing there are problems related to one's own consciousness but there are also issues related to the failure of being a reliable researcher and colleague. Promotion of unfair competition implies cheating upon society which listens to and depends on research in many areas to inform political decisions. If legislation and policies are built on false results, people may be harmed, and if research proves to be unreliable, trust in research decreases, which may lead to less support from both private and public funding bodies (VR, 2011). For all these reasons, if revealed at some point, research based on false results must be retracted (e.g. by publishing a correction in a journal). See Table 1.1 for an overview of examples of scientific misconduct and questionable conduct of research taken from the world of animal research.

I.2 ETHICAL AWARENESS IN DESIGN OF ANIMAL RESEARCH

A central part of responsible conduct of research is how experiments are designed. When designing a study with animals, scientists are

Table 1.1 *Different phases of research and examples of type of misconduct in animal research*

Phase of research	Example of kind of misconduct	Practical example from research with animals
Research setup and design	Not complying with the rules for authorization of animal experiments Lack of implementation of guidelines	Non-compliance with the animal experiment license was found in a published paper; the experiment reported tumour growth beyond what was approved for that experiment. This lead to a published correction and apology by the authors (Nature, 2015; Raj *et al.*, 2015).[a]
Handling of research material	Insufficient responsibility for material Fabrication or falsification of data Plagiarism (misleading use of material, ideas, designs, methods etc.) Lack of implementation of guidelines	Fabrication of data, exemplified by a classical case in 1974 in transplantation immunology: William T. Summerlin fabricated changes in skin colours of mice by painting them with a permanent marker as an evidence of successful transplantation.
Research collaboration incl. authorship	Lack of responsibility for research process, lack of contribution Plagiarism (wrongful appropriation of texts) Order of authors, false or gift authorship, excluded from authorship in spite of substantial contribution	A paper on social stress and pain perception in mice was found to have plagiarized 17 sources. This lead to retraction of the paper (PLoS One, 2016; RetractionWatch, 2016).[b]

(continued)

Table 1.1 *(continued)*

Phase of research	Example of kind of misconduct	Practical example from research with animals
Publishing results	Limitation of 'relevant' results and manipulated results Dishonesty about a person's contribution	A paper on nutritional supplementation methods in sheep production was withdrawn due to complaints about the data presented and the attributions of authorship (RetractionWatch, 2015; Sweeny *et al.*, 2015).[c]

[a] http://www.nature.com/news/protection-priority-1.18354 Correction and excuse by authors: L. Raj *et al. Nature* http://dx.doi.org/10.1038/nature15370; 2015

[b] http://retractionwatch.com/2016/05/31/plos-one-paper-plagiarized-from-17-articles-yes-17/#more-40553. The retraction note: http://journals.plos.org/plosone/article?id=10.1371/journal.pone.0156567

[c] http://retractionwatch.com/2015/08/11/sheep-study-pulled-for-issues-with-the-validity-of-data-and-attribution-of-authorship/#more-30416. The retraction note: http://www.sciencedirect.com/science/article/pii/S1090023315002555

Source: Original table by Röcklinsberg, Gjerris and Olsson.

mainly motivated by the research question they want to address. They are hopefully well acquainted with the present state of the art of methodologies in the field and the questions for which an answer is necessary to move the field forward. The overall plan of research will probably have been presented in an application for funding and its scientific merit evaluated by other scientists. Presently, nearly all scientific research in academia takes place within funded projects which have undergone this kind of scientific evaluation.

In industry, decisions to go ahead with animal experiments will be based on an internal scientific discussion and economic evaluation. For the other main area of animal experiments, the so-called

regulatory testing, it is the legal requirements for testing new substances and devices which provide the reason for using animals. Such
testing uses strictly defined protocols which are applicable across a
range of substances, because all testing basically attempts to answer
the same question: is this substance or device likely to be safe to use
in the way that it is intended? In contrast, research is much more
variable and highly dependent on the field in which it is conducted
and on the questions to be asked.

It takes more than scientific excellence to plan and run a
good research project with animals. Different skills are needed and
represented by different groups of personnel. Selecting an appropriate animal model for the research question requires knowledge
about the biological differences between different animal species
in different respects. To design the experiment properly requires
understanding of experimental design from both the biological
and statistical perspectives. These are competences of the responsible scientist, but other personnel (animal caretakers, technicians, attending veterinarians, research students) also need to be
competent in the tasks they have to carry out in the study. In the
Directive 2010/63/EU four main tasks in animal-based research are
pinpointed and connected to a range of requirements to be fulfilled
in mandatory education of these groups (see Table 1.2). In addition,
the experiments need to be done in appropriate facilities to produce
reliable results.

I.3 RELATION BETWEEN RESEARCH ETHICS,
ANIMAL ETHICS AND ANIMAL WELFARE

Well-conducted research may correspond with sincere ethical considerations regarding research ethics. From an ethical point of view,
it is, however, not merely a question of conducting research in a good
way to get the best results, but also of considering the ethical issues
related to the animals themselves. Whereas the main responsibility
for how studies are designed and executed lies with the researcher,
there are also instituted mechanisms to ensure that animal research

Table 1.2 *Proposal of the topics in which different types of personnel must be competent, according to a European Commission expert working group on training*

Topic	Function according to Directive 2010/63/EU Article 23			
	(a) carrying out procedures on animals	(b) designing procedures and projects	(c) taking care of animals; or	(d) killing animals
National legislation	●	●	●	●
Ethics, animal welfare and the 3Rs	●	●	●	●
Basic and appropriate biology	○	●	○	○
Animal care, health and management	●	●	●	●
Recognition of pain, suffering and distress	●	●	●	●
Humane methods of killing	●	●	●	● ○
Minimally invasive procedures	● ○	●	●	●
Design of procedures and projects		●		

● theoretical competence ○ practical skills

Source: EWG, 2014.

complies with basic expectations of society. There is of course a variety of views on how or even if animals can be used in research, and different ethical theories give support to different positions. For example, if one shares a radical animal rights view, all medical research for the sake of humans will be unjustifiable, whereas other positions allow for use of animals but with different limitations or constraints regarding impairment of animal welfare (see Chapter 2 for more detailed discussion). A kind of a compromise position underpins legislation saying that animal research is acceptable only when there are no alternative methods to achieve the objective; when animal suffering and animal numbers are minimized; and when the harms caused to animals are justified by the expected benefit of the research. In most countries, one important mechanism to ensure compliance is to require that projects involving use of animals are reviewed before they can start. Usually this review is carried out by a group of people with different backgrounds – often called an Animal Ethics Committee or an Animal Care and Use Committee.

This, however, raises further questions, specifically regarding the definition of harm, as there is no general agreement on what constitutes a harm. Also, 'minimized animal numbers' needs to be explored in relation to statistical parameters to justify the use of them in the first place. It is the task of both researcher and ethical committee to balance potential benefits to humans and possible welfare impairments for the animals. Such a balancing process requires acquaintance not only with research procedures and practices but also with different parameters and measurements relevant in welfare assessment, as well as familiarity with considerations of animal and research ethics. Each decision by an animal ethics committee can thus be seen as a meeting point for issues of animal ethics, research ethics, animal welfare and research design (see Figure 1.1).

Another example of the interdependence of these fields concerns how to handle risks in animal research. The consequences of some procedures on animals are difficult to predict. Parameters to consider are whether the risks are large or small, whether they occur

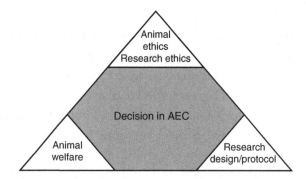

FIGURE 1.1 Three distinct fields of research, each contributing with necessary perspectives on research procedures, here exemplified with the different aspects contributing to a decision of an Animal Ethics Committee (AEC). They are also interdependent, as a decision in any of the disciplines influences what issues are evoked or questions posed in the others, and hence also the outcome of what is deemed ethically justifiable.

Source: Original figure by Röcklinsberg, Gjerris and Olsson.

frequently or seldom, are direct or indirect, as well as easy or difficult to detect. The best approach then is to consider such procedures through a risk assessment, in which one considers the potential harmful consequences, the likelihood that they will occur and measures to be taken not to cause more harm than necessary. The creation of a new line of genetically modified animals is a good example of a procedure with a welfare risk until the phenotype of the animals has been characterized and its effect on their welfare is known (Turgeon and Meloche, 2009).

Experiments using stressed or otherwise impaired animals will in most procedures produce results different from the ones using animals that are better off. Moreover, from a research ethics point of view, if the animal welfare status is not known at the outset, it is difficult to evaluate whether the welfare status influences the results, and thus the results will be difficult to interpret. Further, if complications are not known, e.g. a mouse is infected with a contagious disease without clinical symptoms, this might have an unnoticed impact on the animal. In such instances, researchers will not only evaluate results based on insufficient knowledge, but the ethical evaluation will be flawed as well. Unpredictable or unknown changes in animal welfare might cause unpredictable or unknown effects on the animal and influence results without the researcher's knowledge.

To put it more positively, sincere research ethical considerations will help with choosing a relevant research question, finding the most suitable methodology and producing trustworthy interpretation of results. In animal-based research, research ethical considerations include awareness of the importance of good animal housing and handling for accurate and relevant results. Reliable research results thus are dependent on both well-handled animals and researchers' personal engagement in research ethical dimensions of their work.

I.4   ETHICAL REASONING IN ANIMAL ETHICS COMMITTEES

Given that ethical reasoning is beneficial for the research community, for the animals and for research as such, and hence important, how then is ethics understood by researchers and committee members? There are only a few studies describing this. According to a German study by Kolar and Ruhdel (2007) Animal Ethics Committee (AEC) members had disparate experiences of how an ethical evaluation was performed. The majority performed their own ethical evaluation (42 of 52), whereas fewer relied on the applicants' statements if comprehensive (10 of 52), and 3 out of 52 referred to the ethics discussions in the committee and another 3 found ethical considerations were entirely lacking in the committee work. This latter group consisted of animal welfare representatives.

In a study by Ideland (2009) on ethical reasoning in animal ethics committees in Sweden, informants expressed different views on what the term 'ethics' meant for them in their committee work. Furthermore, when asked for whose sake they were doing this, three clearly different reasons were presented. The answer of the scientists was 'for the sake of science', lay persons from political parties (although not representing such) answered 'for the case of patients' and lay persons from animal welfare organizations said 'for the sake

of animals'. These different views were not found to be explicitly discussed during committee meetings, nor was there an effort to reach a
common view. Rather, Ideland could, in line with other studies (e.g.
Sengupta and Lo, 2003; Tjärnström, 2013) see an established hier-
archy in the committee, where scientists' statements and perspectives set the agenda.

> Even if the scientific experts are not in the majority, they have
> power over the agenda. Observations from the committee
> meetings show that the priority of interpretation belongs –
> exclusively – to scientific ideals. There is no room for ethical
> questions about research purposes and animal suffering in this
> context. (Ideland, 2009, p. 260)

One obvious explanation for the predominance of scientific ideals is
that the entire activity lies within their arena. Another is the traditional perception among scientifically trained persons of science as
objective and ethics as subjective. The believed value neutrality of
science is widely disputed, however (Rollin, 2006; see also Chapter 2),
and the discipline of ethics strives for solid coherent argumentation
as the basis for justification of a position, and thereby can be seen as
intersubjective. An ethical evaluation of a research application builds
on considering relevant facts and an ethical evaluation of these facts
(e.g. considering welfare definition and justification of minimum
welfare levels) but also taking general issues of human responsibility
for humans and animals into account. In this latter aspect emotions
and empathy have a role to play.

Interesting enough, scientists and lay persons' perception
seem to differ when it comes to the role of emotions and empathy.
According to recent studies of Swedish AECs (Tjärnström, 2013),
lay persons decide to exclude emotions from the discussion for tac-
tical reasons. Scientists, who have the leading role during meetings,
instead argue that in order to ensure rationality and objectivity in
the decisions, emotions should be excluded. Taking research on ethical discernments in animal ethics into account, one could, however,

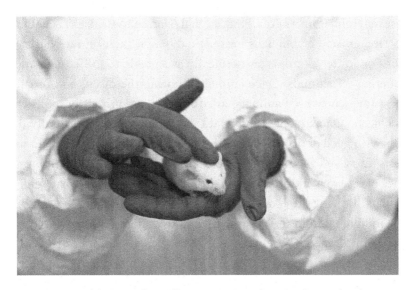

FIGURE 1.2 Need for empathy within science, in order to understand and interpret the welfare situation of the animal.

Source: Image © Understanding Animal Research, www.understandinganimal research.org.uk.

argue that considering the cognitive dimension of emotions would actually be useful in the deliberation (Figure 1.2). Also, the very basis for legislation on use of animals in research is the concern for their welfare, which in turn is based on the scientifically based assumption that animal experiences of pain, stress etc. are relevantly similar to ours (Broom, 2011). Every evaluation of what is regarded an acceptable level of suffering implies that we have access to understand what this suffering, albeit by analogy, means for the animals concerned.

This leads to the issue of how scientists and technicians actually perceive and relate to research animals. Since the late 1980s sociological studies have been performed on this subject (e.g. Birke *et al.*, 2007; Holmberg, 2008; Lynch, 1988). They found that scientists and technicians, knowing they handle sentient beings, changed their perception of the animal as they worked within the area of animal research: from a subject to an object, from having feelings to being a research tool, from a naturalistic animal to an analytical tool. That is, researchers and technicians formulate different kinds of rationalizations or strategies to make it ethically acceptable to inflict pain and suffering on animals. Once animals (limiting the discussion to the most frequently used animals, mice and rats) are primarily regarded as objects. One strategy to uphold this distance to them as individuals with good or bad welfare is to stress the connotation to them as pests, dirty and vectors of disease, another to stress the high importance of research, a third to distinguish between 'good' and 'bad' individuals allowing the good ones to be treated better, and even exclude one individual from the experiment and treat it as a pet.

Simultaneously there is a need to keep a 'feeling for the animal', as this facilitates better care and research results (Holmberg, 2008). This balance between objectifying (in order to be emotionally able and ethically allowed to perform research) and empathy (in order to take good care of the animal) is difficult. One tool to handle this potential moral stress in good balance is through ongoing ethical reflection in the research team, including animal caretakers. Consensus is unlikely to be reached, but elaboration on own reactions and feelings regarding value clashes between e.g. animal welfare and human needs, laboratory traditions or legislation, may facilitate balancing of pros and cons and lead to a way of handling moral stress. Further, when formulation of standardization of procedures and applying good laboratory practice builds on reflection on a practice, it may contribute to continuous discussion of ethical aspects such as e.g. level of acceptable suffering and stress. The difficult task of each researcher, technician and committee member is to decide what is necessary, without becoming cynical while balancing the view of the animal between sentient animal and instrument.

QUESTIONS FOR DISCUSSION AND REFLECTION

1. What considerations should go into designing an animal experiment from a scientific and an ethical perspective respectively?

2. What risks are relevant to look at when designing an animal experiment?
3. How can the relationship between scientific objectivity and empathy to the animals used in research be understood?

REFERENCES

Birke, L.I., Arluke, A. & Michael, M. (2007). *The sacrifice: How scientific experiments transform animals and people*. West Lafayette, IN: Purdue University Press.

Broom, D.M. (2011). A history of animal welfare science. *Acta Biotheoretica*, 59: 121–137.

European Science Foundation (ESF). (2011). *The European Code of Conduct for Research Integrity*. http://ec.europa.eu/research/participants/data/ref/h2020/other/hi/h2020-ethics_code-of-conduct_en.pdf (accessed 12 December 2016).

Expert Working Group (EWG). (2014). Expert Working Group to develop a common education and training framework EC. A working document on the development of a common education and training framework to fulfil the requirements under the Directive. http://ec.europa.eu/environment/chemicals/lab_animals/pdf/Endorsed_E-T.pdf (accessed 12 December 2016).

Holmberg, T. (2008). A feeling for the animal: On becoming an experimentalist. *Society & Animals*, 16: 316–335.

Ideland, M. (2009). Different views on ethics: How animal ethics is situated in a committee culture. *Journal of Medical Ethics*, 35: 258–261.

Kolar, R. & Ruhdel, I. (2007). A survey concerning the work of ethics committees and licensing authorities for animal experiments in Germany. *ALTEX*, 24: 326–334.

Lynch, M.E. (1988). Sacrifice and the transformation of the animal body into a scientific object: Laboratory culture and ritual practice in the neurosciences. *Social Studies of Science*, 18: 265–289.

Ministry of Higher Education and Science. (2014). *Danish Code of Conduct for Research Integrity*. http://ufm.dk/publikationer/2014/the-danish-code-of-conduct-for-research-integrity (accessed 17 February 2017).

Nature. (2015). Protection priority: All involved in animal research must ensure that rules for ethical experiments are observed. *Nature*, 525: 290.

PloS One. (2016). Retraction: The effect of social stress on chronic pain perception in female and male mice. *PLoS ONE*, 11: e0156567.

Raj, L. Ide, T. Gurkar, A.U. Foley, M. Schenone, M, Li, X. Tolliday, N.J. Golub, T.R. Carr, A.A. Shamji, A.F. Stern, A.M. Mandinova, A. Schreiber, S.L. & Lee,

S.W. (2015). Corrigendum: Selective killing of cancer cells by a small molecule targeting the stress response to ROS. *Nature*, 526: 596.

RetractionWatch. (2015). Sheep study pulled for issues with 'the validity of data' and 'attribution of authorship'. http://retractionwatch.com/2015/08/11/sheep-study-pulled-for-issues-with-the-validity-of-data-and-attribution-of-authorship/#more-30416 (accessed 12 December 2016).

RetractionWatch. (2016). PLOS ONE paper plagiarized from 17 articles – yes, 17. http://retractionwatch.com/2016/05/31/plos-one-paper-plagiarized-from-17-articles-yes-17/#more-40553 (accessed 12 December 2016).

Rollin, B.E. (2006). The regulation of animal research and the emergence of animal ethics: A conceptual history. *Theoretical Medicine and Bioethics*, 27: 285–304.

Sengupta, S. & Lo, B. (2003). The roles and experiences of nonaffiliated and non-scientist members of institutional review boards. *Academic Medicine*, 78: 212–218.

Sweeny, J.P.A. Surridge, V. Humphry, P.S. Pugh, H. & Mamo, K. (2015). Retraction notice to 'Benefits of different urea supplementation methods on the production performances of Merino sheep' [*The Veterinary Journal* 200 (2014) 398–403]. *The Veterinary Journal* 206, 118.

Tjärnström, E. (2013). *Decision making and the role of empathy in animal ethics committees (AECs)*. Swedish University of Agricultural Sciences. Department of Animal Environment and Health (MSc Thesis 2013:503) http://stud.epsilon.slu.se/6325/1/Tjarnstrom_E_131216.pdf

Turgeon, B. Meloche, S. (2009). Interpreting neonatal lethal phenotypes in mouse mutants: Insights into gene function and human diseases. *Physiological Reviews*, 89: 1–26.

VR (The Swedish Research Council). (2011). *Good Research Practice*. Vetenskapsrådets Rapportserie, vol 3:2011.

2   The Ethical Perspective

To obtain valid results from research involving living animals, both scientific skills and a good understanding of the animals are needed. That the science is conducted in a good way and gives valuable results does not, however, in itself answer the ethical question: *Should we do research on living animals*?

From certain ethical perspectives the answer is a resounding: 'yes!' Humans can perhaps benefit from this research, and animals are just animals. If we can help humans, we should use animals as the resources they are. Seen through other ethical perspectives, animals matter more and the research needs to be justified by weighing the pain, stress, discomfort and suffering imposed on the animals against the benefits that the research can lead to. Still others outright reject that humans can use animals for research, claiming that we have no right to sacrifice them for our own purposes. To others, again, the answer becomes a question of how humans should relate to animals to become authentic humans.

All these different answers rest on basic assumptions about the human-animal relationship: what the intrinsic values of humans and animals are and how humans ought to use the power that we, by help of our rationality and technology, have in relation to animals. The differing positions on these issues lead to the often heated debates on the ethics of using animals for research. In this chapter we discuss what ethics is and present an overview of the most important ethical positions in the ethical debate on research animals.

2.1   WHAT IS MORALITY AND ETHICS?

When we experience the world, we experience what takes place through a filter of values that help us to discern whether what takes place is right or wrong. This evaluation is based on deep-seated values that we often, at least in the situation, are not even consciously aware of. If I see a person being attacked on the street for no apparent reason, I might wonder whether I have the courage to interfere and how best to do it – but I do not wonder whether it is right or wrong that s/he is being attacked. Later it might turn out that s/he was attacked because s/he was threatening other people with a concealed weapon, and I therefore have reason to change my initial evaluation of the situation. But that does not change that most of us usually are very quick to form an opinion on the ethical aspects of a situation. Moral reactions are thus an integrated part of our way of responding to the world and based on deep-seated values about how the world ought to be. It is on the basis of these values that the world around evokes in us emotions of approval or rejection (Gjerris *et al.*, 2013, pp. 1–10).

As shown earlier, we cannot always rely on our immediate feelings. We might not have all the relevant facts, or we might have misunderstood the situation and thus come to change our opinion when the facts become clearer to us. Or we might find ourselves in a situation where we experience that there are several values at stake at the same time and be unsure as to which of them carries (or carry) the most weight for us. This is where our initial moral reaction ought to lead us to ethical reflection, where we begin to evaluate the situation based on our understanding of the facts and an understanding of the involved values and their importance. Our morality, formed by a certain social, cultural and religious context, is deeply connected to our feelings and inform us that something seems to be either right or wrong. Ethics, on the other hand, is what takes place when we do not just rely on these emotions, but critically reflect on them. Ethics is thus a philosophical reflection on morality. Although different ethical positions have different views on the role of emotions for ethical decisions, it is generally acknowledged that emotions have a crucial role in establishing an ethical awareness. On the one hand, emotions are subjective, and might be easy to dismiss by anyone who strives for objective evaluations. On the other hand, morality heavily relies on empathy and emotions. Although no one can ever feel exactly what another being feels, the similarities between us are numerous enough that we often take for granted that we can obtain an informed idea about how others are faring. Without empathy we could not even grasp what another person's situation means for that person, e.g. how it feels to be hurt, or share the joy of a good meal or companionship. By excluding emotions or empathy we would reduce our ethical capacity to make balanced decisions, as emotions are involved in a number of cognitive processes such as problem solving, learning ability and social evaluations.

According to both research on decision-making processes in ethical issues (Haidt, 2001; Mencl and May, 2009; Pizarro, 2000) and research about how to think in ethical terms in the first place (Diamond, 1983; Nussbaum, 2001), emotions and empathy play a crucial role. Empathy for others gives an important basis for understanding their situation and motivates us to act in a decent way towards them. In the next step, making decisions how to act, emotions and empathy shape our perception and what to focus. A study by Mencl and May (2009) showed that

> [a]s empathy and a sense of responsibility for others increase, focus on costs and benefits of the outcome of a certain situation decreases, meaning that empathy can be said to be more closely linked with virtue-based ethics rather than with principle-based ethics. When there is less emotional attachment and identification, the decision-maker is more prone to focusing on the outcomes rather than the responsibilities of a situation, implying that a more utilitarian ethical approach is expected. (Tjärnström, 2013)

Following this research, we should consider letting emotion and reason be mutually active in a 'personal equilibrium' in each ethical decision (Callahan, 1988; see also Nussbaum, 2001).

In the following we give an introduction to ethical issues evoked by animal-based research (Section 2.2), and thereafter present a number of ethical theories (Section 2.3). While doing so, we proceed from those ascribing emotions a nihilist or limited role to those ascribing a more substantial role by starting with principlist theories such as utilitarianism and rights theory and proceed via virtue ethics to feminist ethics of care.

2.2   ANIMAL RESEARCH ETHICS

Ethics raises very general questions about how we ought to live with other human beings, animals and nature. But it also raises more specialized questions within the different spheres of human life. One such sphere is animal research, where both people working within the field and people on the outside often have strong opinions. This is hardly a surprise, as two very widespread and deeply held values that are difficult to combine clash here. The first is that we – all things being equal – ought to alleviate human suffering. The other is that we – all things being equal – ought to treat animals in a good way. It is hardly a surprise that there are strong disagreements as to how this trade-off should be done – or if it should be done at all.

Animal research is not only done to improve human health and alleviate human suffering; it is also done for a variety of reasons such as improving efficiency in food production, understanding how to treat or prevent animal diseases and zoonoses, or as basic research to understand such things as metabolism. Animals are not always subjected to intensive suffering in the experiments. Some experiments rely mainly on observation and others on only minor interventions in the lives of the animals – besides the obvious caging or housing. Nonetheless the paradigmatic case of animal research in ethical terms is often seen as the trade-off between human welfare and lives or between animal welfare and lives, and has been extensively discussed by ethicists (Nordgren, 2010).

The importance of animal research for human health is evaluated by opponents to animal use as wildly exaggerated (PETA, 2015), but is described by others as indispensable for almost any progress in medicine (Understanding Animal Research, 2015; see Section 3.5 for a thorough discussion of this issue). This kind of factual disagreement can be hard to resolve, as it can be difficult to agree on how to measure the importance of animal research for human health. Even harder are the more value-laden disagreements on whether it is justifiable at all to use animals, and *if* so, when. Often the factual and ethical disagreements blend together and the different interpretations of the factual knowledge seem to be dependent on the values held by the interpreters. However, there are certain basic ethical values that clearly divide the participants in the debates. In the following section we describe some of these. First of all we need to ask the very basic question: Does an animal matter in any ethical sense?

2.3 WHO AND WHAT IS ETHICALLY RELEVANT?

Who or what is ethically relevant in itself and thereby sets ethical limits for our use of it as a resource? From an ethical perspective this question can be approached by dividing everything in the universe into three categories depending on how their moral status is conceived: ethical agents, ethical subjects and ethical objects.

Ethical agents are the ones that act in the situation – hence the name *agent*. They are beings that it makes sense to hold responsible for their actions. They understand that there is a difference between right and wrong and have some ability to at least partially predict the outcome of their actions. Ethical agents are in short beings we would deem fit to stand trial for their actions. They are ethically responsible for others and expected to be able to shoulder this responsibility – or understand that they have failed. At the same time, they deserve ethical treatment themselves from other ethical agents. Being an ethical agent means that you have both obligations and rights.

Ethical subjects are beings considered ethically relevant in themselves. The agent acts on behalf of the ethical subject, taking its interests and intrinsic value into consideration, not his or her own – hence the name *subject*. Ethical agents are, as mentioned earlier, themselves a subgroup within the group of ethical subjects. But most of us will agree that there are ethical subjects who do not have the capacities of ethical agents. Small children and the severely mentally disabled are not considered responsible for their actions in the way adults such as the readers of this book are. Nonetheless, most will still claim that small children and the severely mentally disabled have an ethical importance in themselves and cannot be treated at the whim of ethical agents.

Ethical objects are the kind of beings and things that ethical agents are not directly responsible for. They are, however, not irrelevant, as the way the agents interact with them might have a negative or positive influence on ethical agents or subjects – hence the name *object*. If I borrow a phone from my friend and then loose it, I am responsible for my friend's loss – but not for the phone itself. I have not wronged the phone, as there is, morally speaking, nothing to wrong in a phone, but I have wronged my friend. Ethical objects might thus have huge indirect importance, as they can influence ethical agents and subjects, but they do not have ethical importance in themselves (Gjerris *et al.*, 2013, pp. 49–51).

Turning to the ethics of animal research, it becomes rather important to decide which category animals belong to. Even though it is debated whether some animals can exhibit at least rudimentary moral behaviour (Bekoff and Pierce, 2009), the crucial question in this regard is whether animals should be seen as ethical subjects or objects. If they are ethical subjects, they put quite different moral demands on us than if we regard them as merely ethical objects. Not surprisingly, different answers exist to this question. In the following section we will present the most prominent ethical theories related to animal research and see how they answer this and other questions related to the ethical relationship between humans and animals.

2.4   ETHICAL THEORIES AND ANIMAL RESEARCH

Ethics has always been part of human existence. Even the oldest known oral and written traditions contain explicit values related to humans, states and gods. As an academic discipline in the Western tradition, the roots of modern ethics is often traced back to the classical Greece and philosophers like Plato (428/427–348/347 BC) and his most famous pupil, Aristotle (384–322 BC). A range of ethical theories has been developed in the time span from then until today. Ethical theories differ from scientific theories in that they try to say something about not only how the world is (descriptive) but also how it should be (normative). A normative ethical theory is thus, in the discipline of ethics and in the context of this book, an attempt to show which values are the most important and why it is so.

There is one important distinction to make here between two different issues within ethical reasoning. One concerns the question from the previous section *who or what is an object of moral concern?* (Who is ethically relevant?) Related questions are whether all (beings or entities) that are relevant are equally relevant or if some, e.g. humans, are more relevant than others, e.g. animals? Further, what phenomena are ethically important to protect – life, freedom or welfare? Ideally all three are relevant, but how to prioritize them, if that becomes necessary?

The second issue concerns *what constitutes an ethically justified action.* Different answers are suggested within different *normative ethical theories.* They seek to systematize the cacophony of values and principles that we encounter in our everyday discussions as humans and professionals. By doing this we gain more clarity of the complexity of the issues and the involved values. But often the individual can have a hard time identifying with just one of the theories. Most of us can relate to several of them and use them interchangeably depending on the issue and the context. It is not a failure if one is not able to react to all cases according to one certain normative theory, e.g. as a full-blood contractarian or deontologist. An example of how hard it can be to 'belong' to just one position can be seen and tried out in the online educational tool 'Animal Ethics Dilemma' (2016). We suggest theories should rather be seen as tools to understand the discussion than tools to make the ethical decisions for us. That said, there is still a need to aim for consistency (internal logic) and well-argued points of departure in one's ethical views.

In what follows we present a number of ethical theories that provide different answers to the questions mentioned earlier and therefore can help illuminate the ethical debates on animal research – and provide an answer to the main question of this chapter: *Should we do research on living animals*? It should be mentioned that there are other theories and various versions out there. We have chosen the ones we believe are most central to the discussions on the ethics of research animals today and which, taken together, reflect the width of normative ideas surrounding the issue. Needless to say, the depth of these theories cannot be presented here; the aim is to give an understanding of the different viewpoints. If the reader should wish for more in-depth knowledge about the theories, we recommend using the literature referred to in this chapter.

2.4.1 *Contractarianism*

Contractarianism begins with the simple question: Why should I act in an ethical manner? Even though there can be a lot of disagreement on what exactly is meant by 'ethical manner', most will probably agree that not stealing, being trustworthy, helpful and in general behaving within the norms of contemporary society is part of acting in an 'ethical manner'. But why should we do so? The contractarian answer is very simple: 'You should do so because it benefits... yourself'.

Contractarianism was most clearly formulated as an ethical theory by the British philosopher Thomas Hobbes (1588–1679) who in his book *Leviathan* from 1651 argued that by accepting common rules and a sovereign ruler each individual would be better off than if each just was to fend for him- or herself. Contractarianism, also known as *social contract theory*, thus bases the relationship between humans on self-interest. As long as you gain more than you lose from working together with others and adhering to the common rules, you should do so, as it will lead to the best results for you.

Ethics thus becomes prudence. 'What's in it for me?' is the basic question with the caveat that often there is more in it for you, if you consider that your actions will affect the help and support others will grant you. But – importantly – if you can get away with e.g. breaking a promise and come out the richer even in the long run, then there is no obligation for you to honour the original contract. You do, how-ever, have to remember that your gain might cost you in the long run if it leads others to disrespect the social contract as well.

This way of looking at ethics carries with it the implication that the only beings you need to treat according to the common rules are those that have the ability to understand and react negatively to you, if you do not stay within the limits of the social contract. They are, so to speak, the only ethical subjects – remembering that to the contractar-ian only the own person is actually relevant. The consideration towards the others only goes as far as reflected self-interest (prudence) goes. One can say that they end up being a kind of active ethical objects.

Animals cannot enter into a social contract. To the contractar-ian they are therefore nothing but means to reach his or her ends. It is a bad idea to mistreat your neighbour's dog, not because it would wrong the dog, but because you could lose social goodwill in relation to your neighbour. This has clear implications for the contractarian view on using animals in research. The animal simply does not exist as anything but a tool to gain advantages for the contractarian e.g. in the medical area. At the same time, however, the contractarian has to take into account the economic, emotional, social etc. effects that can come out of using animals in research. Will it in the end lead to the best life possible for the contractarian – or will it have more nega-tive than positive consequences?

One can thus not say whether the contractarian will be positive or negative to the use of animals in research in general. It depends on an evaluation of the specific situation taking into account all the possible consequences for the contractarian. What can be said very clearly, however, is that the animals are not important in themselves, i.e. are not regarded as moral subjects. As long as the contractarian finds him- or herself gaining from it, anything can basically be done to animals. As the philosopher Jan Narveson writes,

> On the one hand, humans have nothing generally to gain by
> voluntarily refraining from (for instance) killing animals or

'treating them as mere means'. And on the other, animals cannot generally make agreements with us anyway, even if we wanted to have them do so. (Narveson, 1983, p. 58)

2.4.2 *Utilitarianism*

Utilitarianism is the idea that from an ethical viewpoint our actions should not be directed towards our own good, but towards maximizing the common good. This overall good can for the utilitarian briefly be said to be the quality of life for all those that can experience quality of life or, to state it even more briefly, welfare. There are obviously many discussions on how to define quality of life or welfare more precisely. To the English lawyer Jeremy Bentham (1748–1832), who is one of the founders of utilitarianism, welfare was closely connected to hedonism – a theory focusing on the mental experiences of individuals no matter the source. The focus was on subjective mental experiences of pleasure/joy and pain/suffering. The task was to maximize the overall welfare of all beings capable of experiencing such mental states. This view famously led Bentham to include animals in the ethical community as ethical subjects: as their welfare could be better and worse, they mattered ethically. As Bentham wrote: 'The question is not, Can they reason? nor Can they talk? but, Can they suffer?' (Bentham, 2007, chapter XVII, note 122).

Besides maximizing the overall welfare of all concerned, Bentham suggested two other principles that should govern moral actions. One concerns the question of moral concern and is called the *principle of equality*. Everyone's interests are equally important, which was a very radical statement those days. There are thus no moral grounds from which one can claim that one's own welfare is more important than that of others. Moreover, Bentham argued this principle should be applied also to animals, i.e. the welfare of mice and men counts equally in the cost-gain calculation to maximize the overall good. Obviously we have different interests and humans are usually considered to have a higher capability for suffering than mice. But if e.g. a mouse stands to lose more welfare than I would in a given situation, the fact that I am a human or just plain self-interest cannot be used as a justification to forego the welfare of the mouse. Hence, if it would, all things being equal, maximize the overall welfare if I promote the welfare of the mouse instead of my own, this is the correct action to opt for.

The second important principle presented by Bentham is that the welfare of some ethical subjects can be sacrificed as long as it can be argued convincingly that it will increase the overall welfare. In this sense utilitarianism can be seen as the philosophical equivalent to the old saying: *The end justifies the means.* Utilitarianism is therefore also known as a consequentialist theory. It is only the consequences of an action as they relate to welfare that are interesting to evaluate. The motives are not important in themselves; what counts are what positive or negative consequences they have. If we turn to the use of animals in research, it becomes clear that the underlying ethical rationale in modern-day biomedical animal experimentation is largely utilitarian in nature. We cause (to varying degrees) pain and suffering in some beings (animals) to achieve knowledge that can help us prevent or alleviate pain and suffering in other beings (humans) in the hope of thereby maximizing the overall welfare.

The most well-known philosopher within contemporary animal ethics is the Australian Peter Singer, who since the 1970s has written extensively on animal ethics from a utilitarian perspective. Singer famously has promoted including animals into the ethical community, arguing that not doing so would be speciesism. First put forth by the British animal rights activist Richard Ryder in 1970, this argument claims that distinguishing between the ethical importance of humans and animals simply based on species membership is parallel to racism or sexism, as species membership (just as gender or ethnic origin) is ethically irrelevant. Rather, what is ethically relevant, both Singer and Ryder argue, is the ability of both humans and some animals to experience suffering and joy.

One of Singer's contributions has been to qualify the idea of welfare as put forward by Bentham by arguing that what counts for a being is to have its preferences fulfilled. Thus when figuring out how to maximize the welfare, the idea is that one should aim to satisfy as many preferences as possible while taking into account that the welfare following the fulfilment will vary in relation to the importance of the preference for the individual. Satisfying a crucial preference for one being thus might be better than satisfying the trivial preference of several beings. Singer further discriminates between basic and other needs, the former referring to e.g. food and water, shelter, social interactions and the latter to all other needs, including luxury food, mink coats, driving a certain car etc. In the balancing between needs one should primarily satisfy the basic need of all relevant beings before satisfying other needs of anybody (Singer, 1975).

Thus, the utilitarian position contains ways to justify at least some use of animals for human purposes, but it also presents huge challenges. Here we discuss just the most important elements as they relate to the question of using animals in research. From a philosophical viewpoint, many more could be discussed, e.g. when a preference is legitimate and whether welfare is really all that matters – how about *truth* in itself for example? For a discussion of these matters we refer you to the general introduction to ethics by Gjerris *et al.* (2013).

The utilitarian position allows for animal research as long as the outcome can convincingly be shown to lead to the greatest overall welfare. This is in line with what many people believe regarding use of animals. Thus only few would protest if inflicting pain or suffering on mice could help to alleviate the mental losses experienced by Alzheimer patients. On the other hand, this is exactly where the challenges pop up, because how do we compare the actual pain and suffering of the mice to the possibility that the research performed might end up helping humans? In theory, utilitarianism seems clear and almost mathematical in its weighing pros and cons and deciding for the optimal outcome. The problems occur as soon as the situation becomes just a little complex. What should count as pros and cons? How much weight should we put on them? How do we assess what amount of welfare gain and welfare loss is produced during a given research procedure and how do we compare it? How can we fairly estimate the positive outcome of e.g. basic research into the metabolism of rabbits and compare it to the loss of the rabbits?

The utilitarian judgement thus rests on many preconceptions of different aspects of the total outcome, which the theory itself cannot give an answer to. That is, there will not be only one possible answer following from a utilitarian analysis. For example: How much weight should we assign to the positive experiences arising from eating bacon compared to the welfare levels of pigs in intensive production systems, the effects of the production on environment, climate, economy, human health etc.? To be able to discuss whether a certain research project involving animals is justifiable from a utilitarian perspective, it is very important that there is as much transparency as possible about the research in itself, the likelihood that it will lead to increased welfare for other beings later in the process, what consequences one has taken into the welfare estimation etc.

Utilitarianism thus both brings the animals into the ethical community as ethical subjects and at the same time allows for their welfare and lives to be sacrificed, if it can be argued that it will maximize the overall welfare. An interesting point to leave you with is that in being true to the principle of equality, the theory implies the same for humans. If no side constraints are built into the theory, humans can also be sacrificed as long as it can be shown to maximize the overall welfare.

2.4.3 Theories on Animal Rights

The idea that animals can have moral rights in a similar way as humans has grown out of the philosophical tradition known as *deontology*. The most renowned thinker within this tradition is the German philosopher Immanuel Kant (1724–1804), although he himself reserved the status of ethical subjects to humans. Kant's thinking was very influential in the development that led to the Universal Declaration on Human Rights that was adopted by the United Nations General Assembly in 1948 (UN, 1948). Based on the criteria of rationality, Kant argued that only humans are objects of direct moral concern. All rational beings that have the ability to understand moral obligations have an intrinsic value that grants them certain inalienable rights such as liberty, equality and independence. The perhaps most famous formulation of Kant on the subject of duties is:

> Act in such a way that you treat humanity, whether in your
> own person or in the person of any other, always at the same
> time as an end and never merely as a means to an end. (Kant and
> Ellington, 1993, p. 30)

Latching on to this tradition, a number of philosophers has sought to expand the circle of right holders (beings that should always be treated as an end in themselves) to include animals. The most influential of these is undoubtedly the American philosopher Tom Regan (1938-2017), who in continued discussion with Peter Singer since the 1970s has developed an animal rights theory. There are other theories within this tradition, but for the sake of clarity we have chosen to present only Regan's thoughts here.

Three questions are necessary to answer, when one claims that animals can have moral rights in analogy to humans: (1) Which animals have rights? (2) Why do they have rights? (3) What rights do they have? Regan's answer to the first question – i.e. who is a moral subject – is that all animals that can be characterized as a *subject-of-a-life* have rights. Regan defines *subject-of-a-life* as beings that

> have beliefs and desires; perception, memory, and a sense of the
> future, including their own future; an emotional life together
> with feelings of pleasure and pain; preference – and welfare –
> interests; the ability to initiate action in pursuit of their desires
> and goals; a psychophysical identity over time; and an individual
> welfare in the sense that their experiential life fares well or ill for
> them, logically independently of their being the object of anyone
> else's interests. (Regan, 1987, p. 243)

A subject-of-a-life thus has preference interests, i.e. an interest in what happens to it. Hence a rat has preference interests, but a stone does not. Precisely which animals are capable of this will have to be decided in biological studies of each kind of animal to determine if it lives up to the demands listed above – much as the utilitarian relies on scientific facts about which animals can experience welfare or which cannot. For our purposes here we simply state that for now vertebrates and cephalopods are among such animals (which are included in the Directive 2010/63/EU as objects of concern). Whether e.g. certain types of insects can be said to be subjects-of-a-life or experience welfare is still debated (see e.g. Gjerris *et al.*, 2016). It is worth noting that Regan does not build his argument on attribution of moral status to the ability to feel better or worse (welfare), but to the ability to have preferences: beliefs, desires, goals. Based on these characteristics, the ethical community of beings that should always be treated *as an end and never merely as a means to an end* (see discussion of Kant earlier in the chapter) according to Regan includes not merely rational human beings but at least some non-human animals –those having the aforementioned beliefs, desires and goals.

The basic right that follows from Regan's thinking is that these animals should be treated with respect. They should be allowed to pursue their own end and not be used as instruments by humans to reach ends that are irrelevant to them. Only when the two coincide and humans can reach a desired end without interfering in the attempts of the animal to fulfil its own desires and beliefs can it be said that the animals have been treated with respect. Adopting this view will have radical consequences and is often labelled *abolitionist* by those adhering to it, referring back to the movement against slavery beginning in the late eighteenth century. Both within research, food production, the entertainment industry and the pet industry most uses of animals would have to cease. On the question of using animals in research, Regan writes:

> In the case of the use of animals in science, the rights view is
> categorically abolitionist ... these animals are treated routinely,

> systematically as if their value were reducible to their usefulness
> to others, they are routinely, systematically treated with a lack
> of respect, and thus are their rights routinely, systematically
> violated. It is not just refinement or reduction that is called
> for, not just larger, cleaner cages, not just more generous use of
> anesthetic or the elimination of multiple surgery, not just tidying
> up the system. It is complete replacement. The best we can do...
> is – not to use them. That is where our duty lies, according to the
> rights view. (Regan, 1985, p. 25)

The consequences of Regan's position are unacceptable to some as it abolishes the whole idea of using animals for human purposes in almost all situations. More moderate versions of animal rights theories have therefore been developed, often combining some basic rights with a utilitarian approach. One noteworthy example of such an approach is *The Five Freedoms* that grew out of the criticism of intensive farm animal production by e.g. Ruth Harrison (1964) in Britain in the early 1960s and the subsequent work of the Brambell Committee and later the British Farm Animal Welfare Council. Focusing on farm animals, *The Five Freedoms* were formulated thus: (1) freedom from hunger and thirst; (2) freedom from discomfort; (3) freedom from pain, injury and disease; (4) freedom to express (most) normal behaviour; and (5) freedom from fear and distress (Vapnek and Chapman, 2010). Two basic 'freedoms' that would be obvious to grant the animals within the thinking of Regan are missing, namely the freedom to act on your preferences and the freedom not to be killed for ends that are not your own.

Moreover, it is obvious that *The Five Freedoms* only to some degree is relevant for research animals, as some of the freedoms are incompatible with doing certain types of research. For example, it is hard to perform research on drugs that remove or alleviate pain if you cannot inflict pain on the animal to begin with. But the compromise between the radical rights approach and the utilitarian approach is also present in the world of research animals. Thus the

EU Directive (2010/63/EU) on the Protection of Animals Used for Scientific Purposes states:

> (23) From an ethical standpoint, there should be an upper limit of pain, suffering and distress above which animals should not be subjected in scientific procedures. To that end, the performance of procedures that result in severe pain, suffering or distress, which is likely to be long-lasting and cannot be ameliorated, should be prohibited. (European Commission, 2010; see also Chapter 5.2.)

This shows the same balance between rights and utility of which *The Five Freedoms* is an expression. Animals can be used for human ends, but there is an upper limit for what they can be subjected to. There is little doubt that the discussion between what can be labelled strong and weak animal rights positions will continue in the future. The EU legislation sets the long-term goal of abolishing the use of animals in research as soon as there are alternatives that can provide the same quality research, whereas in the meantime it sets limits to how animals can be treated. Thus, one might say that for pragmatic reasons the legislation now mirrors the weak animal rights position combined with an utilitarian weighing of the best outcome, while the long-time aspirations are more in line with the view of the strong animal rights position.

2.4.4 *Virtue Ethics*

Virtue ethics is classified as a normative ethical theory, but compared with utilitarianism and deontology, it does not ask for one norm or criteria to discern whether an act or intention is ethically justifiable. Rather, a virtue ethics approach to moral issues takes its point of departure in the question 'how to be a good person?'. This shall not be understood as a self-centred question, but shifts the focus from certain norms (to follow) to the character of the person acting: 'How shall I behave in order to act as a virtuous person in this specific situation?'. Hence, virtue ethics focuses on the ethical agent, and is context sensitive, i.e. relates its discernment to the actual situation.

However, not any self-made ideas on what is a good character will do. According to Aristotle (384–322 BC) who formulated the most well known of the early writings on virtue ethics, there is a set of virtues to guide one's action. While personal responsibility to grasp ethical issues at stake in each context is crucial, as well as formation of one's character, core virtues are defined in and by the community (or praxis). Aristotle distinguishes between moral and intellectual virtues. The most important of the moral virtues are the so-called cardinal virtues: prudence, justice, fortitude and temperance. Each of these virtues, and others such as courage and friendship, have opposites that should be avoided. According to Aristotle, our task is to find the golden middle way. For example, a courageous person is neither reckless nor a coward. The intellectual virtues are related to our capacity to evaluate a situation (synesis), and to our practical reason (phronesis) enabling us both to know about the good life and to discern how to act in each situation. The ideal of good life shall not be understood in terms of wealth or material goods, although poverty is no ideal, but rather to intellectual freedom and wisdom, which in turn leads to happiness (eudemonia).

In order to become a true virtuous person, these virtues should be incorporated in one's character and become an internal part of oneself. A virtuous person strives not to limit the good of others and to internalize a generous, friendly and just behaviour so that this becomes one's spontaneous reaction and action. This should be seen in relation to Aristotle's basic idea of life. Everything has a good, a meaning (telos) and strives to fulfil its potential, 'to become what one is'. He even speaks of 'realising the divine in each human' (Bartlett and Collins, 2011). Thanks to our rationality, humans have more capacities than other living beings and a higher moral status, but other living beings also strive to reach their potential and, if so, are 'flourishing'. Denying a bird to fly or a mouse to build a nest would hence be to restrict its possibility to flourish, whereas a human developing its emotional and intellectual capacity can be said to flourish.

Virtues are formulated within a community (praxis), but there is room for interpretation. A virtue might have a slightly different meaning for different persons, as situations are understood on basis of previous experiences (what someone intend as just might be perceived as unjust by someone else). Differences which are not fundamental, but rather those of a degree, are not a big problem within virtue ethics, as the idea is that everybody acts according to own discernment and understanding of what is responsible.

Seen from the position of other normative theories, this lack of clear answers and judgement of what is an ethically correct action and what is not can be criticized. On the other hand, virtue ethicists can claim that they seek to base their decisions on an informed understanding of the actual situation and the virtues needed to make life flourish, and openly put forth their arguments to be criticized. In this they are not any guiltier of the lack of clarity than ethicists coming from different positions. Moral agents following a consequentialist theory need to make a judgement of what aspects to include in a calculation and how to balance pros and cons, whereas a deontologist needs to discern what the relevant universal components are in a certain context to make a relevant judgement of what duty to follow or what right to respect. The demand for ethical theories to deliver clear and unambiguous answers might simply be an expression of a misunderstanding of what ethics actually is about.

There are a few well-known virtue ethicists working on animal issues, such as Martha Nussbaum and Rosalind Hursthouse, but they do not address the use of animals in research to the same extent as proponents for utilitarianism and animal rights theories have done. Hursthouse (2006) argues that the idea of moral status is not useful for a virtue ethicist, as the question of how to distinguish between moral subjects and moral objects is not helpful to guide actions. Rather, we shall consider what character trait we want to inherit and what practice we want to be a part of. Considering medical research and industry, it is, she states, realistic to say that changing it would be hard. The question is what kind of world one wants to participate in creating, and our responsibility is related to the position one has. That is, certain roles are connected to certain virtues, leading to legitimate expectations from others. For example, a project leader may well strive to be inspiring and just, whereas the co-workers strive to be conscientious and trustworthy. From a virtue ethics point of view, then, each researcher designing a study and each technician in the lab has to consider how s/he as a responsible person can take animal and human suffering as well as probability of success into account. Hence, depending on how previous experiences and evaluation of the situation (synesis) are combined in practical wisdom (phronesis), different virtue ethicists may advocate more or less restrictive approaches to animal-based research.

An example of what a virtue ethics approach can lead to can be found in a paper by Cheryl Abatte. She argues that a minimally decent animal ethic requires a framework that allows for context-dependent considerations of our complex human–animal relationship in a non-ideal world. She sees virtue ethics as a theory that enables society to balance between just maximizing welfare or sticking to a rigid rights framework in relation to animals. This will e.g. enable researchers to justify doing research on animals when vital interests are at stake (cancer research), but closing down the opportunity if it is for more trivial purposes (hair loss), even though this could maximize welfare from a utilitarian viewpoint (Abbate, 2014). Abatte's position has similarities with Anders Nordgren's, who formulates a middle position between radically against and uncritically positive use if animals in research. He too argues for case-by-case judgements, but stress the need of imaginative casuistry (Nordgren, 2010). Imagination enables us to take suffering of both animals and humans into account, and our moral capacity helps us to discern and see relevant aspects in each case. The most suitable starting point for a sincere evaluation of animal use is, he argues, the question: 'What should be done if our children or grandchildren suffer from this or that disease?' (Nordgren, 2010, p. 82). Nordgren's answer is that one should take all persons that can be said to have an interest in a particular kind of research into account, and then evaluate the research by solid discernment of human and animal interests, welfare, concepts of rights, animal integrity, interspecies integrity etc.

2.4.5   *Feminist Theories on Animal Ethics*

Feminist ethics has its roots in late eighteenth-century argumentation for emancipation and equal rights by activists such as Mary Wollstonecraft (1759–1797). It cannot be described only as an ethical theory, since it also has political dimensions and builds on sociological studies and descriptions of injustices in society. Hence, it aims in its very core to change the situation of women by increasing equality between women and men at all levels by criticizing e.g. traditional patriarchal dualisms used (e.g. men vs. women, reason vs. emotion). Today, one of the most influential feminist approaches is ethics of care, which stresses interdependence and responsibility rather than rights or calculation of utility. This is not only a shift in focus from whom to entitle rights, or how to evaluate the goods, but also a point of departure more similar to virtue ethics. Since the 1980s, ethics of care has been developed to include animals (mainly concerning issues in holding animals at farms, in labs, circuses, zoos and as companion animals). A number of different versions have been developed (Donovan and Adams, 2007), and in the following the key traits of feminist ethics of care are described.

In feminist ethics of care animals are regarded as sentient individuals with feelings that humans can identify with, and who are largely dependent of human action for their welfare. This calls for human responsibility and an obligation to consider animals' individual needs as related to species and personalities. Hence attention to the individual animal is a core commitment. Attention further applies to the causes of impaired animal welfare, i.e. also scrutiny of ideological, political and financial systems preserving hierarchies and discrimination. Similar to animal ethicists from other normative theories, it is argued that a higher level of transparency regarding how animals are treated is a prerequisite for change. However, different from utilitarians and animal rights theorists, feminist ethics (in similarity with virtue ethics) criticize the idea of pinpointing certain qualities or capacities required for moral status and rights.

From this feminist perspective, a focus on rights is not seen as relevant, since it rests on the flawed idea of a necessary similarity between humans and animals both in general and with respect to autonomy and rationality. Further, it is an expression of a flawed understanding of what a society is: It falsely considers society to be built on independent beings and has difficulties motivating care for non-autonomous beings. Rather, both humans and animals are interdependent, and care for all in need is crucial. Another problem is that a focus on rights largely excludes emotions as relevant for morality, although it is well known to be a basis for moral motivation. Finally the rights perspective is seen as too abstract because of the focus on formal and universal principles (just as in utilitarianism). Rather, feminist thinkers claim that moral discernment requires attention to the context and the particularities of those affected. In this last point one can see obvious similarities with virtue ethics.

Due to this situational approach and avoidance of principles other than showing attendance, there are no outspoken guidelines in terms of a general order of principles. This is potentially a difficulty when care for human health requires use of animals in research. There is no universal principle against interaction or holding domestic animals, but through the focus on attention to the individual and its entitlement to being taken care of on own premises, it is open for interpretation whether instrumentalization is prohibited or not. Is it acceptable to use animals if they are well taken care of until dead? Or does attention to individual animals always require no use at all for human purposes?

A strict version can be formulated in which no use of animals for human purposes can be justified if this implies impaired welfare at any stage. Taking mice as an example, breeding practices, housing in standard cages and even non-invasive procedures reduce the welfare compared to a possible situation offering natural mating, nest-building, care of offspring and unlimited space and social interaction, and hence cannot be justified. This reasoning builds on a fundamental idea in ethics that it is relevant to distinguish between active and passive action, and hence from such a strict version it makes a difference whether we as humans cause welfare loss or whether the mice have impaired welfare due to living their lives in the wild.

In a less strict version, very good housing facilities meeting species-specific and personality-related needs of each individual mouse would be acceptable. If followed by painless killing, post-mortem use could even be positively evaluated given it contributes to better human health or welfare.

2.4.6   Core Differences between the Theories When Applied to Animal Research

Finally we elaborate on some core differences between these theories using some practical examples, the first being killing, or euthanasia as it is often labelled in a lab animal context. Within several ethical theories, respect for the animal as such, not only what it experiences in terms of impaired welfare, is considered relevant. If one considers, for example, animals to basically have a right to a good life, the acceptable level of pain inflicted is probably set lower than if one holds the view that animals are resources for human purposes. Causing death is problematic from an animal rights position, whereas the act of killing is ethically neutral in a utilitarian view. Here only the level of suffering inflicted compared to the outcome matters.

A utilitarian researcher needs knowledge about the particular situation, but a crucial difference from e.g. a virtue ethical inspired researcher is that s/he does not strive to be a good person through his or her acts, but rather to maximize the overall welfare. If this can be reached only by exposing animals to extreme pain and suffering, one should still perform the act, whereas a virtue ethicist could resist based on considering what it is to be a good person and what practices one agrees with (Gjerris *et al.*, 2013) (see also Section 4.2).

Such context sensitivity calls for knowledge about what a certain species, or even individual, is expected to experience at the outset of an experiment (e.g. genetic modification, breeding practice, housing system). Further, such an experiment should be seen from an animal welfare point of view (e.g. injection or sampling method, location and frequency, effect of triggering a genetic defect or housing in metabolic cages). Depending on the choice of welfare definition (see Section 3.2), different aspects come to the fore. It is up to the researcher to argue whether primarily health, subjective experiences or natural behaviour should be taken into consideration, and why not all three are given the same weight, when assessing the animal welfare at stake.

QUESTIONS FOR DISCUSSION AND REFLECTION

1. What is the role of ethics in discussions on how animals are used and housed in research and how their welfare is affected?
2. What are the possibilities and challenges related to ethical thinking when designing animal experiments?
3. Describe the basic differences between (a) a utilitarian and a virtue ethics position, and (b) between an animal rights and an ethics-of-care position.
4. What is the value of analysing research on animals by looking at it from different ethical perspectives?

REFERENCES

Abbate, C. (2014). Virtues and animals: A minimally decent ethic for practical living in a non-ideal world. *Journal of Agricultural and Environmental Ethics*, 27: 909–929.

Animal Ethics Dilemma. http://www.aedilemma.net/ (accessed 12 December 2016).

Bartlett, R.C. & Collins, S.D. (2011). *Aristotle's Nicomachean ethics*. Chicago: University of Chicago Press.

Bekoff, M. & Pierce, J. (2009). *Wild justice: The moral lives of animals*. Chicago: University of Chicago Press.

Bentham, J. (2007). *An introduction to the principles of morals and legislation*. New York: Courier Corporation.

Callahan, S. (1988). The role of emotion in ethical decisionmaking. *Hastings Center Report*, 18: 9–14.

Diamond, C. (1983). Having a rough story about what moral philosophy is. *New Literary History*, 15: 155–169.

Donovan, J. & Adams, C. (2007). *The feminist care tradition in animal ethics: A reader*. New York: Columbia University Press.

European Commission. (2010). Directive 2010/63/EU on the protection of animals used for scientific purposes. Official Journal of the European Union. L276: 33–79. http://eur-lex.europa.eu/LexUriServ/LexUriServ.do?uri=OJ:L:2010:276:00 33:0079:en:pdf (accessed 12 December 2016).

Gjerris, M. Nielsen, M.E.J. & Sandøe, P. (2013). *The good, the right & the fair: An introduction to ethics*. London: College Publications.

Gjerris, M. Gamborg, C. & Röcklinsberg, H. (2016). Ethical aspects of insect production for food and feed. *Journal of Insects as Food and Feed*, 2: 101–110.

Haidt, J. (2001). The emotional dog and its rational tail: A social intuitionist approach to moral judgment. *Psychological Review*, 108: 814–834.

Harrison, R. (1964). *Animal machines: The new factory farming industry*. London: Vincent Stuart Publishers.

Hursthouse, R. (2006). Applying virtue ethics to our treatment of the other animals. In J. Welchman (ed.), *The practice of virtue: Classic and contemporary readings in virtue ethics*. Indianapolis, Hackett Publishing Company, pp. 136–154.

Kant, I. & Ellington, J.W. (1993). *Grounding for the metaphysics of morals: With on a supposed right to lie because of philanthropic concerns*. Indianapolis, IN: Hackett Publishing.

Mencl, J. & May, D.R. (2009). The effects of proximity and empathy on ethical decision-making: An exploratory investigation. *Journal of Business Ethics*, 85: 201–226.

Narveson, J. (1983). Animal rights revisited. In H.B. Miller & W.H. Williams (eds.), *Ethics and animals*. New York: Springer, pp. 45–59.

Nordgren, A. (2010). *For our children: The ethics of animal experimentation in the age of genetic engineering, vol 215*. Amsterdam: Rodopi.

Nussbaum, M. (2001). *The intelligence of emotions*. New York: Cambridge University Press.

People for the Ethical Treatment of Animals (PETA). (2015). Animal Testing 101. http://www.peta.org/issues/animals-used-for-experimentation (accessed 12 February 2015).

Pizarro, D. (2000). Nothing more than feelings? The role of emotions in moral judgment. *Journal for the Theory of Social Behaviour*, 30: 355–375.

Regan, T. (1985). The case for animal rights. In P. Singer (ed.), *In defense of animals*. New York: Basil Blackwell, pp. 13–26.

(1987). *The case for animal rights*. New York: Springer.

Singer, P. (1975). *Animal liberation*. New York: Harper Collins.

Tjärnström, E. (2013). *Decision making and the role of empathy in animal ethics committees (AECs)*. MSc thesis, Swedish University of Agricultural Sciences.

Understanding Animal Research. (2015). Human Health. http://www.understanding animalresearch.org.uk/why/human-health (accessed 12 February 2015).

United Nations (UN). (1948). Universal Declaration on Human Rights. http://www.un.org/en/documents/udhr/index.shtml (accessed 12 December 2016).

Vapnek, J. & Chapman, M. (2010). *Legislative and regulatory options for animal welfare*. Rome: Food and Agriculture Organization of the United Nations.

3   The 3Rs and Good Scientific Practice

With Catarina Vieira de Castro

In this chapter, we give an introduction to the use of animals in research. We discuss how research may negatively affect animal welfare and how such harm to animals can be reduced. We also address the scientific relevance of research and discuss issues in translational research, i.e. how to ensure scientific relevance of research with animals. Further, examples of relevant guidelines and recommendations are included and discussed.

3.1   HOW ARE ANIMALS USED IN RESEARCH?

Studies on living animals play an important role when seeking to find new knowledge, developing applications such as drugs and in testing the safety of new substances and devices. Research represents the largest single proportion of animal use in experiments in most recent European statistics (European Commission, 2013b). A large proportion of this research falls into the biomedical category, where animals are studied to understand the functioning of the body and the mechanisms involved in the diseases that affect it (*basic* biomedical research) or used to develop and test therapies for such diseases (*applied* biomedical research). The ultimate goal of both lines of research is commonly to extrapolate results to the human case. When animals are used as models of human diseases, the research implies to induce in them conditions which, at least in some aspects, mimic the conditions that researchers aim to understand in humans and for which they wish to develop appropriate treatment. Most animals

This chapter is partly based on a previously published book chapter, Vieira de Castro, A.C. and I.A.S Olsson (2015), *Does the goal justify the methods? Harm and benefit in neuroscience research using animals*. Curr Top Behav Neurosci, **19**: p. 47-78.

used in biomedical research are of the typical laboratory animal species: rats, mice and, to an increasing extent, zebrafish. Laboratory animals are also used in basic biology research (for example, to understand the function of different genes), where again they are mainly studied as models of something, in this case a biological function. In contrast, in agricultural and veterinary research, animals are often studied to find out things like more effective feeding regimes or better disease treatments for other animals of the same species.

The use of animals for research remains a controversial issue. The main controversy lies in the fact that most research is done for human benefit and the animals are often harmed by the research, which they cannot consent to participate in. Not surprisingly, animal experimentation has been challenged primarily on grounds of animal suffering for nearly as long as animals have been used in research (see Franco, 2013 for an overview). That the controversy is well and alive today was clearly evident in the turbulent discussions accompanying the revision of European legislation leading up to Directive 2010/63/EU (see subsection 5.2.1). Within a year of its transposition into national legislation, the directive was challenged by a citizen's initiative urging 'the European Commission to abrogate Directive 2010/63/EU on the protection of animals used for scientific purposes and to present a new proposal that does away with animal experimentation' (EurActiv, 2013). On the other side of this debate there are movements defending the importance of continued access to animal research as a way of answering important biomedical questions, and more specifically a statement in support of the present legislation signed by more than a hundred research institutions, companies, learned societies and non-governmental organizations (NGOs) (WellcomeTrust, 2016).

Experiments often require housing the animals under restrictive and stressful conditions, and different degrees of physical or psychological harm can result from protocols which are used to induce diseases mimicking the human diseases under study. Distressing or painful interventions may be part of experimental protocols.

Harm to animals includes adverse effects on health, as well as all the adverse subjective experiences animals might undergo, such as pain, fear or anxiety. The end of the research usually implies the end of the life of the laboratory animals, at least in the case of mice and rats (larger animals are usually kept for longer periods of time and used in repeated experiments). We also regard such killing as a harm, based on the understanding that killing will only be in the animal's own best interest in cases of severe conditions from which recovery is not possible and where there is substantial suffering which cannot be relieved otherwise. For most research animals in most situations, life presents both positive and negative experiences, and killing an animal will prevent it from all potential future positive experiences (Yeates, 2010).

One special field of ethical concerns is related to genetic modification of animals used for research. In general there are two kinds of concerns, the first related to the modification as such, questioning our right to change the genetic make-up of another individual. This argument is frequent in relation to farm animals or plants, but rarely raised in the context of laboratory animals and will not be discussed further here. A second cluster of concerns is related to the consequences for the actual animals – in particular in terms of poor welfare of animals born with or developing defects. For already existing genetically modified strains, these consequences are known, whereas the generation of new lines requires a prediction of negative effects and a strategy for dealing with them. These issues are usually considered as part of assessing animal harm.

3.2 ANIMAL HARM AND ANIMAL WELFARE:
WHAT IS IT AND HOW CAN IT BE ASSESSED?

In the first section of this chapter, we gave some examples of harm inflicted on animals in experimental research. The harms exemplified in the previous section include effects on animal health but also adverse subjective experiences resulting from the experimental interventions. Health and subjective experiences both form part of what is commonly understood to represent 'animal welfare', and considerable research is directed towards understanding how animal welfare is affected by internal and external factors, as well as towards developing methods for assessing welfare status or changes to welfare.

Animal welfare is a broad concept, although how broadly it is defined varies somewhat among sources. In their seminal text, animal welfare professors Ian Duncan and David Fraser highlight three main approaches: one focussing on subjective experiences (feelings), one focussing on biological functioning (health) and one focussing on the nature of the animals (Duncan and Fraser, 1997). Official definitions such as that of the World Organization for Animal Health (OIE) tend to include at least the subjective feelings and the biological functioning approaches:

> Animal welfare means how an animal is coping with the conditions in which it lives. An animal is in a good state of welfare if (as indicated by scientific evidence) it is healthy, comfortable, well nourished, safe, able to express innate behaviour, and if it is not suffering from unpleasant states such as pain, fear and distress. Good animal welfare requires disease prevention and veterinary treatment, appropriate shelter, management, nutrition, humane handling and human slaughter/killing. Animal welfare refers to the state of the animal; the treatment that an animal receives is covered by other terms such as animal care, animal husbandry, and humane treatment. (OIE, 2014)

Reliably measuring the welfare of animals in different situations is important for many activities, including the development of legislation and guidelines. The commonly used animal welfare measures are often divided into two main groups: behavioural and physiological parameters. Behavioural measures include indicators of negative experiences (e.g. pain and fear), time budget changes (e.g. reduced grooming or eating), appearance of abnormal behaviours, and also reaction in specific behaviour tests such as those of preference, motivation and cognitive bias. Physiological measures include indicators of health and of stress (Olsson, 2010).

Translating animal welfare research into ways of assessing animal welfare in practical situations require ways of integrating different parameters into one or several aggregate measures, as well as the development of assessment protocols. These challenges were addressed for farm animals through the WelfareQuality® project, proposing that welfare assessment should primarily be done using animal-based parameters and rely on four welfare principles: good housing, good feeding, good health and appropriate behaviour. Spangenberg and Keeling (2016) have proposed an assessment protocol for laboratory animals based on the WelfareQuality® approach. Table 3.1 presents the criteria and assessment parameters they suggest to use.

Animal research ethics committees often have to make predictions about animal welfare. The expected harm to animals to be caused by the procedures is considered during the ethical evaluation of a proposed study. Towards this, guidelines and policy documents for the evaluation of animal experiments have suggested lists of criteria to be assessed in such predictions. These criteria usually include the quality of the facilities, the experience of the personnel caring for and carrying out the procedures on animals, the number of animals, the animal species, the husbandry and housing conditions, the scientific procedures themselves (including the killing method), considering the duration and the intensity of the pain or distress likely to be inflicted on the animal, the fate of the animals at the end of the experiments and the endpoints to be applied (e.g. APC, 2003; Smith and Boyd, 1991; Smith et al., 2007).

Some regulatory systems further ask for an assessment of the severity of procedures or experiments, that is, the degree of pain or suffering likely to be experienced by animals. In assessing the negative impact on the animal, the duration and frequency of a procedure is considered. As illustrations, Table 3.2 presents the severity classifications adopted by the European Union in Directive 2010/63/EU and by the Canadian Council on Animal Care (CCAC). The EU

Table 3.1 *Criteria and assessment parameters for a welfare protocol for laboratory animals based on the WelfareQuality® approach as suggested by Spangenberg and Keeling.*

Welfare principles	Welfare criteria	Mouse parameters
Good feeding	Absence of prolonged hunger	Body condition Ability to reach the food hopper (CCP at weaning)
	Absence of prolonged thirst	Dehydration Ability to reach the water nipple (CCP at weaning)
Good housing	Comfort around resting Thermal comfort Ease of movement	Nest building performance Pups outside the nest Gait/movements
Good health	Absence of injuries	Lameness Piloerection Hunched position Wounds (excluding bite wounds)
	Absence of diseases	Urine and faeces Coat condition Ocular/nasal discharge Distended abdomen Other deviations (innate/acquired)
	Absence of pain induced by management procedures	Activity and interaction with environment Facial expressions of pain
Appropriate behaviour	Expression of social behaviours	Whisker and/or fur trimming Bite wounds/marks Vocalizations/audible fights in cage Blood stains in cage
	Expression of other behaviours	Circling Jumping against cage wall Bar chewing
	Good human-animal relationship	Approaching hand in cage Ease of handling when moving mice from dirty to clean cage Urination/defecation during handling
	Positive emotional states	Rearing

CCP: critical control point.

Source: Spangenberg and Keeling (2016).

Table 3.2 *Severity classifications of animal experiments from the European Directive 63/2010/EU (left column) and the Canadian Council on Animal Care (CCAC, 1991, middle column) illustrating the different categories (right column).*

EU Directive	CCAC Guidelines	Examples
Non-recovery Procedures which are performed entirely under general anaesthesia from which the animal shall not recover consciousness	Included under **B**	
	A Experiments on most invertebrates or live isolates	The use of tissue culture and tissues obtained at necropsy or from the slaughterhouse; the use of invertebrates
	B Experiments which cause little or no discomfort or stress	Short restraint for observation or physical examination; blood sampling; injection of non-irritating substances in small amounts; acute non-recovery studies; approved methods of euthanasia; short food / water deprivation equivalent to natural situations.

(continued)

Table 3.2 (*continued*)

EU Directive	CCAC Guidelines	Examples
Mild Procedures on animals as a result of which the animals are likely to experience short-term mild pain, suffering or distress, as well as procedures with no significant impairment of the well-being or general condition of the animals	**C** Experiments which cause minor stress or pain of short duration	Cannulation, catheterization and minor surgery under anaesthesia; short food / water deprivation exceeding natural situations; behavioural experiments with short-term, stressful restraint; exposure to non-lethal levels of drugs or chemicals. Tumours with no adverse effects; breeding of genetically altered animals of mild phenotypes; diets that do not fully meet nutritional needs
Moderate Procedures on animals as a result of which the animals are likely to experience short-term moderate pain, suffering or distress, or long-lasting mild pain, suffering or distress as well as procedures that are likely to cause moderate impairment of the well-being or general condition of the animals	**D** Experiments which cause moderate to severe distress or discomfort	Major surgery under general anaesthesia with subsequent recovery; prolonged physical restraint; behavioural stress induction; procedures which cause severe, persistent sensorimotor disruption; the use of Freund's Complete Adjuvant. Models of tumours causing moderate pain or distress; irradiation or chemotherapy with a sublethal dose with mild/moderate and short-lived adverse effects; breeding of genetically altered animals of moderate phenotypes;

Severe		
Procedures on animals as a result of which the animals are likely to experience severe pain, suffering or distress, or long-lasting moderate pain, suffering or distress as well as procedures, that are likely to cause severe impairment of the well-being or general condition of the animals	**E** Procedures which cause severe pain near, at, or above the pain tolerance threshold of unanaesthetized conscious animals	Testing of substances/devices leading to severe pain, distress or death; vaccine potency testing with persistent impairment of the animal's condition, progressive disease (including tumours) with long-lasting moderate pain, distress or suffering leading to death; irradiation or chemotherapy with a lethal dose; inescapable electric shock; prolonged complete isolation of social species.
		Exposure to noxious stimuli or agents with unknown effects; exposure to drugs or chemicals at levels causing death, severe pain, or extreme distress; completely new biomedical experiments which have a high degree of invasiveness; behavioural studies with unknown effects; use of muscle relaxants or paralytic drugs without anaesthetics; burn or trauma infliction on unanaesthetized animals; euthanasia with non-approved methods not approved by the CCAC; any procedures resulting in unrelieved pain which approaches the pain tolerance threshold.

Source: Original table by Castro, Röcklinsberg, Gjerris and Olsson.

Directive requires that experiments are attributed a severity classification (non-recovery, mild, moderate or severe) determined by the degree of pain, suffering, distress or lasting harm expected to be experienced by an individual animal during the course of the procedure. For more than 20 years, evaluation under the CCAC has applied a similar scale of 'Categories of Invasiveness in Animal Experiments' ranging from experiments on most invertebrates or on live isolates (A) to procedures in vertebrates and some invertebrates which may cause severe pain (E) (CCAC, 1991). Protocols must be submitted to an appropriate review committee for all studies which involve the use of vertebrates and some invertebrates in Categories B through E. Both the European Directive and the CCAC guidelines give potential examples of experimental procedures which are considered to be representative of each category.

In addition, individual procedures are often combined within an experiment, and the nature of each procedure is not the only factor determining severity. How large the impact on the individual animal is will further be influenced by biological characteristics determined by species, strain and genotype and previous experience of the animals. Animals differ in sensitivity to different interventions because of mental as well as physical characteristics. A more fearful animal will be more affected by restraint and manipulation than a calmer animal will. Many physical interventions are more invasive in smaller animals than in larger animals. Factors of relevance for impact, related with the procedures, include if the procedure is surgical or not, how strongly and for how long animals are restrained, whether it is painful and if pain control is provided and whether other refinements are applied. In addition, issues having to do with frequency, repetition of procedure and total accumulated experience of the animal have to be considered. This is not straightforward, since repetition may result in habituation and therefore reduce severity, or it may result in increased severity if causing animals to anticipate a stressful procedure or increase pain sensitivity (European Commission, 2012). The examples given in European legislation and Canadian guidelines

(Table 3.2) provide some concrete examples of different severity categories. However, they are generally limited in scope and provide little guidance as to how to consider total impact resulting from a combination of different procedures. Therefore, animal ethics committees often rely primarily on their own collective experience and best judgement when performing the comprehensive assessment of degree of severity of animal harm which is part of the evaluation of research proposals. In this process, the extended welfare assessment grid proposed by animal welfare scientists Paul Honess and Sarah Wolfensohn (2010) may be useful. This approach brings together a range of parameters indicating the welfare of research animals into one single entity, which can be illustrated graphically. Figure 3.1 shows an example of how the lifetime experience of a laboratory macaque changes with its use in a vaccination study.

Whereas much of the discussion focuses on the impact of procedures the animals are subject to, and pathologies they develop as a consequence of research, it is important to keep in mind that laboratory animal welfare is also influenced by how the animals are housed. This issue is also addressed in legislation, obviously through the specific technical regulations of minimum dimension of the animals living space, but also through more general provisions. Directive 2010/63/EU prescribes that animal facilities should be constructed to provide an environment where animals' physiological and ethological needs have been taken into account. It also specifically prescribes that this environment must be sufficiently complex to allow a wide range of behaviours, and further for animals to have some control over their environment. In addition, animals of social species must be kept in social groups of compatible animals. There may, however, be situations when the conditions of research require exceptions. The most common exception is probably when individual housing is the only way to collect important data or avoid that other animals manipulate and pull out surgical implants such as catheters or electrodes. Environmental complexity may need to be reduced temporarily to allow measurements to be taken in metabolic cages.

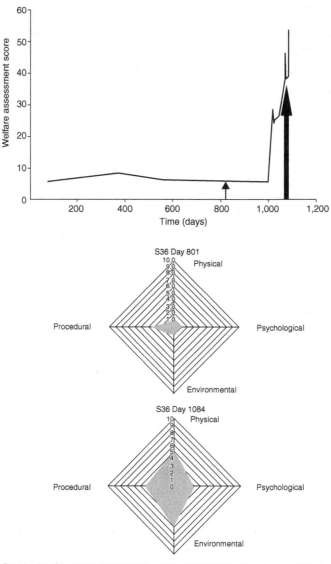

Combined welfare assessment score through animal S36's life (study 3 unvaccinated).

FIGURE 3.1 The animal welfare assessment grid is a way to integrate all experiences of a laboratory animal into a visual illustration. This particular grid illustrates the lifetime experience of a rhesus macaque in a vaccination challenge trial. This particular animal belonged to the unvaccinated control group, and so as a consequence of being infected around day 802 it developed the disease, resulting in a substantial loss of animal welfare starting around day 1,000.

Source: Wolfensohn *et al.* (2015).

Such limitations will have an impact on animal welfare, and the approaches for animal welfare measurement presented in this chapter (the WelfareQuality® approach and the animal welfare assessment grid) are designed to integrate effects of procedures, pathologies and effects of housing. Genetic modifications which lead to pathologies or impairments also need to be taken into consideration in assessing the overall impact of research on animal welfare.

3.3 MINIMIZING ANIMAL HARM: THE 3RS

According to the approach on which animal experimentation is generally based, for an animal experiment to be ethically acceptable, the expected benefits of the research not only must outweigh potential harms, but the harms caused to the animals must be minimized as well: in other words, animals must not endure unnecessary suffering. The 3Rs (Replacement with non-animal methods; Reduction of the number of animals used; Refinement of methods to protect animal welfare), proposed by Russell and Burch (1959), are widely recognized principles in the attempt to minimize harms to animals and, hence, to perform ethically acceptable research. The order of the 3Rs is not arbitrary. First we should ask if the use of animals can be replaced by non-animal methods. Only after determining that animal research is actually needed does it make sense to ask how the number of animals can be reduced and how the research can be refined to minimize animal suffering. Finally, when implementing the principles, the potential impact on research quality also needs to be taken into account.

3.3.1 *Replacing the Use of Animals*

Replacement is the first of the 3Rs, for several reasons:

> Replacement enjoys a particular standing among the 3Rs. It was the first of the Rs to be introduced by Russell and Burch (1959), reflecting the intended order in which the Rs were to be considered. Questions about Reduction and Refinement are only relevant if Replacement has first been considered and excluded.

> The goal of Replacement also has received widespread support, in part because it is the only goal that is fully compatible with the animal rights perspective that animal use solely for human benefit should not be permitted. (Olsson *et al.*, 2011)

The main point of this principle of Replacement is that the use of animals should be replaced by non-animal methods whenever doing so is possible without compromising the research objective. Replacement methods may be in vitro (e.g. cell lines), ex vivo (e.g. tissue cultures) or in silico (e.g. bioinformatics). Often these studies make use of human cells or data from humans, and in fact even research with human volunteers may sometimes be considered as a replacement approach. The idea that studies in human volunteers would be an ethical alternative to the use of animals in research may seem provocative, and it is of course a first prerequisite that such a study meets the ethical standards for research with human subjects – especially that the research subject has provided informed consent. Being able to work with human material rather than with animals of different species is often considered an advantage in that it does not require extrapolation between species.

There are two main limitations of replacement methods. The complexity of the system is reduced when animals are replaced by simpler and more restricted systems, such as cell lines or tissue cultures. In the ethics review (see Section 5.2–5.3), scientists are usually requested to justify why living animals are needed, and the typical answer is that the research question must be studied in an entire living body where all organs are present and in interaction. In studies with human volunteers, the limitations are instead in terms of the kind of interventions which are acceptable, as these cannot jeopardize the long-term health of the study subject. The use of invertebrate animals is sometimes also included within Replacement; Russell and Burch (1959) described this *relative replacement*.

Overall, the greater the role of non-animal methods in research, the fewer animals will be needed in total for research purposes. In this way, replacement is also directly related to the second R: Reduction.

3.3.2 *Reducing Animal Numbers*

The aim with the principle of Reduction is to use the smallest possible number of animals to obtain valid information. Its main ethical purpose is to reduce collective animal harm, understood as the number of animals on which harm is inflicted. One important measure is to use correct and careful statistics, including appropriate power analysis prior to study commencement. Sample sizes can also be decreased by controlling variance associated with different environmental and genetic conditions, as for example, by using uniform housing conditions and inbred animals.

Reduction is probably the most challenging of the 3Rs. There is great political value in bringing down numbers of animals used in experimental procedures as a whole, as the number of animals reported in annual statistics is a very visible and easily understood ethical aspect of use of animals in research. But *how* this reduction is achieved may have great implications for the quality of research. It may be tempting to reduce the number of animals within an experiment. But, as detailed analyses have repeatedly shown, the number of animals used in experiments is often in practice too small for results to be reliable. This of course has important implications for the validity of the research results. Within a larger review of methods in neuroscience, Button *et al.* (2013) examined the statistical power of animal experiments investigating sex differences in water maze and radial maze performance. They found that many studies are underpowered, which means that too few animals were studied for the results to be reliable. This also has ethical consequences (see Section 1.3):

> There is ongoing debate regarding the appropriate balance to strike between using as few animals as possible in experiments and the need to obtain robust, reliable findings. We argue that

it is important to appreciate the waste associated with an underpowered study – even a study that achieves only 80% power still presents a 20% possibility that the animals have been sacrificed without the study detecting the underlying true effect. If the average power in neuroscience animal model studies is between 20–30%, as we observed in our analysis above, the ethical implications are clear.

Low power therefore has an ethical dimension – unreliable research is inefficient and wasteful. This applies to both human and animal research. The principles of the 'three Rs' in animal research (reduce, refine and replace) require appropriate experimental design and statistics – both too many and too few animals present an issue as they reduce the value of research outputs. (Button *et al.*, 2013, pp. 371–372)

Based on this, it does not seem appropriate to apply reduction through decreasing sample sizes in individual experiments as an exclusive measure. To bring down numbers in a study, other approaches in experimental design are needed. This could include the use of imaging techniques allowing the study of disease progress in the same animals rather than in separate groups for separate time points, or greater use of non-animal approaches before moving to an animal model.

3.3.3 *Refining Animal Research*

Whereas the Replacement and Reduction principles reduce harm by avoiding the use of animals, the Refinement principle addresses the welfare of individual animals which are actually used in experiments. This principle states that all experimental procedures shall be adjusted to minimize any pain or discomfort they may cause to the animals. Experiments can be refined in several ways, from the use of anaesthesia and analgesia to control pain, to housing adaptations allowing animals to perform important behaviours and to cater for animals with special needs and the establishment of humane endpoints (at which the experiment is terminated) to prevent or end suffering which cannot be relieved by other measures. Appropriate measures need to be defined for each individual study, taking into account the nature of the harms which need to be mitigated. The scheme for welfare assessment recently proposed by a European working group allows refinement measures to be integrated into the assessment, as illustrated in Table 3.3.

The principle of the 3Rs is already present in much legislation. For example, the European Directive states that 'To ensure that the way in which animals are bred, cared for and used in procedures within the Union is in line with that of the other international and national standards applicable outside the Union, the principles of replacement, reduction and refinement should be considered systematically when implementing this Directive' (Recital no. 11). Although the 3Rs principle was not explicitly referred to in previous European legislation, researchers were asked to use animals only when necessary, to use as few animals as possible and to use procedures having as little impact as possible.

Unfortunately, systematic reviews of the implementation of refinement measures in biomedical research indicate that there is considerable margin for improvement, at least if reporting of research methods in international journals is taken as an indicator of how research is actually done. For example, between 2000 and 2002, pain relief was administered in only around 20% of studies subjecting rodents to potentially painful procedures (Richardson and Flecknell, 2005). In 2009, humane endpoints were only reported in about 20% of studies of mice models of the neurodegenerative disorder Huntington's Disease, with no significant increase in the reporting of this refinement measure during the preceding ten-year period (Franco and Olsson, 2012). There is thus considerable potential for improvement in the area of refinement.

To ensure that research actually delivers the promised benefits is just as ethically important as minimizing harm. This issue is a central topic in animal research, in particular within the context of translation. The background of the concept is that biomedical research is

Table 3.3 *Schematic approach for assessing severity proposed by the European Commission Expert Working Group on severity classification of scientific procedures performed on animals*

Example	What does this study involve doing to the animals?	What will the animals experience? How much suffering might it cause? What might make it worse?	How will suffering be reduced to a minimum?	
		Adverse effects	Methodology and interventions	Endpoints
Genetically-modified SOD1^{G93A} mouse model of ALS		Discomfort associated with motor capacity loss and difficulties to eat, drink and swallow	Housing adaptations (e.g. placing mashed food at a low level and adjusting of bedding to facilitate movement)	Euthanasia of the animals as early as possible in relation to the research goal in order to avoid unnecessary suffering
		Animals may reach complete paralysis		

Bone defects in a surgically induced rat model of osteoporosis	Surgery to create bone defect	Pain and discomfort associated with surgery	Appropriate anaesthesia and analgesia
	Ovariectomy	Pain and discomfort associated with surgery	Appropriate anaesthesia and analgesia
Study of gene function in mammal limb development	Genetically inducing limb malformations	Locomotor impairment	Euthanasia of preterm embryos in order to avoid the birth of malformed animals

Source: Adapted from European Commission. (2013a). Examples to illustrate the process of severity classification, day-to-day assessment and actual severity assessment. http://ec.europa.eu/environment/chemicals/lab_animals/pdf/examples.pdf (accessed January 2017).

done for the purpose of improving human health. Scientific research should generate knowledge about disease mechanisms, which can then be used to develop more effective treatments for these diseases. Therefore, it is important that research results can actually be translated from the laboratory setting to the clinical practice – or from bench-to-bedside as it is expressed in the jargon of translational medicine.

Considerations of how research results translate into practice should in principle be relevant for any situation where the research results have direct or indirect practical application, and are therefore not limited to medicine. If a new feeding regimen is tested on an agricultural research station and found to be effective in preventing diarrhoea in newly weaned piglets, this will only be useful for pig health if similar results are reached when the regimen is applied on actual farms. However, nearly all the discussion of translation takes place in the context of biomedical research with applications to human health, as we will see in the following section.

Basic research is a context in which translation is less of an issue, because this research is done to increase knowledge in general, without having any evident practical use of this knowledge in sight. Although it is assumed that findings are not unique to the species under study, there is generally no need to claim that what is observed in mice should also apply to humans, and if later research shows that mechanisms are indeed different in the two species, this is an additional piece of knowledge rather than a 'problem of translation'. While it is of course equally important that a basic research project uses the best possible experimental design, the question of translation across species is less relevant.

The increased attention to translation derives at least partly from the recognition that there is indeed a problem of translation. More often than desirable, what seems to be a successful treatment in animal studies (preclinical research) does not produce the same effect when tested in humans in clinical studies, the next step in the drug development process. This difficulty in translating apparent therapeutic successes from studies using animals to human clinical trials has received much attention during the last decade. Activists campaigning for the abolition of animal experimentation use examples of translational failures to argue that animal research is useless or even misleading and should therefore be abandoned. Scientists, on the other hand, have tried to understand what underlies translational difficulties and what can be done to overcome them. In the following, we look at some of the main challenges and efforts to improve translation of animal-based research.

3.4   BIOLOGICAL DIFFERENCES BETWEEN SPECIES

On the surface, there are large differences between animals of different species. A mouse has fur and uses legs to walk on the ground, a crow has feathers and uses wings to fly and a salmon has scales and uses fins to swim in water. But research in palaeontology and developmental biology has shown that there are underlying fundamental similarities between these seemingly very different animals. These similarities are explained by the common evolutionary origin of all vertebrate species, and this is what makes scientists able to extrapolate information about biological mechanisms between different species. Nevertheless, this extrapolation is not straightforward and biological differences need to be considered when animals of one species are used to model another species.

Some of the differences between humans and laboratory animals can actually be reduced by changing biological features to make the animals more like humans in aspects which are central for the question under study. This approach has gained importance during the last decade and is primarily applied to mice, which is the most frequently used mammal species in research. The overall idea is to incorporate biological material of human origin into the mouse. This may mean engrafting human cells or tissues into the body of the mouse, where they will function as much as possible like they would do in the human body (Ito *et al.*, 2012). The term 'humanized mice' is sometimes used for mice incorporating human tissue. In immunology, 'humanizing' mice consists in engrafting hematopoietic stem cells into mice which have (nearly) no immune system of their own, and which thereby come to develop a functional immune system which is very similar to that of humans. This means that mice will be susceptible to infectious agents which normally only infect humans, and that therapeutics can be tested to act on human cells (Shultz et al., 2012). Such mice are valuable for research into diseases where the immune system plays an important role. It is also possible to replace the normal microbiota of the mouse intestine by human intestinal microbes, and attempts are being made at making mice with 'human' livers by transplanting human hepatocyte cells to the mouse liver (Ito et al., 2012). Transgenic mice in which a transgene of human origin has been incorporated in the mouse genome, have been used for more than 10 years as models of genetic and other disorders (e.g. Gama Sosa et al., 2012).

Attention to species differences is most important where there is a need to extrapolate directly – as is the case in drug efficacy and toxicology testing. The following statement from a toxicology workshop report explains why it is crucial to understand how and to what extent extrapolation is possible:

> Although experimental animal data often constitute the only available predictor of human health effects, their predictive ability is limited. There are numerous differences between experimental animal and human responses to chemicals, including differences in the types of adverse effects experienced and the dosages at which they occur. The differences may reflect variations in the underlying biochemical mechanisms or in the distribution of the chemicals. It can be expensive or detrimental to public health if experimental animal models are not good predictors of human health effects, so it is critical to select and validate animal models early in the regulatory process. (NRC, 2005: 1–2)

Toxicology and drug efficacy testing are also the only areas where there are explicit standards for which characteristics an animal model should have. These standards are part of the regulatory framework for marketing authorization of pharmaceuticals and chemicals (see e.g. FDA, 2014). However, it is possible to establish similar criteria for animal-based research (see e.g. Varga *et al.*, 2015).

3.5 IMPROVING TRANSLATION

Within the scientific community, there is now a lively discussion of how to ensure that animal research actually delivers its promised benefit of relevant and reliable results. Driving this discussion is the increasing evidence of problems in translating research. Opponents of animal experimentation often use such problems to argue that research with animals should be abandoned altogether. However, the main problem may rather be that many studies with animals are not well designed, something which is of course equally problematic but easier to correct. Most of this knowledge comes from extensive systematic analysis of experimental animal research into stroke. In this field, a wide number of drugs which had proven effective in animal models later failed to work in clinical trials on humans. In many of these experiments, the efficacy of the treatment was probably overestimated as a result of design bias. Often animals were not randomly allocated to treatments, and researchers who were not blinded when they administered the treatment or assessed the outcome, may unconsciously have influenced the measurements (e.g. van der Worp *et al.*, 2005). Similar problems characterize animal research across disciplines (Pound and Bracken, 2014). Thus, more rigorous study methodology is urgent for animal research.

Finally, if the intended benefits of research are to be achieved in practice, the results of the experiments must be made public; hence communication is central. Publication in peer-reviewed journals is a central feature of modern academic research, and, as is well known, the performance of today's researchers is measured largely on the basis of the number of publications they have in influential journals. However, it is generally difficult to get negative results (no effect of treatment) published. As a direct consequence of this, publications are likely to reflect only part of the research that has been carried out in a field – the research in which differences were found between treatment groups. Publication bias, whereby positive results are more likely to be published, has indeed been pointed out as a major problem in research in general (Dwan *et al.*, 2008) as well as research with animals (Sena *et al.*, 2010). It has ethical implications in that it leads to an overestimate of the treatment effects under study and in that animals may be used in vain as studies which have not been reported are repeated by researchers who are unaware that the study had already been done.

Given the problems in translating results from preclinical research with animals to human clinical trials, some attempts have been made to bring researchers together to discuss how to do preclinical research in a given field in the best way (Katz *et al.*, 2012). The major barriers to translational success identified in these workshops were a lack of rigorous standards and transparency in reporting preclinical studies. The subsequent published guidelines from these groups outline some of the principles and standards of good study design and report when conducting preclinical trials of candidate therapeutics – e.g. allocation concealment, blinded assessment of outcome, random allocation of subjects to experimental groups and other methods designed to minimize bias and Type 1 ('false positive') errors.

By raising standards and awareness, these initiatives strive to increase the reliability, reproducibility and predictive value of preclinical research, and ultimately improve the likelihood of success on clinical translation. More attention also seems to be needed to improve the validity of animal models themselves. Finally, publication of negative findings from well-conceived and performed studies should be encouraged. It can help investigators to evaluate and ultimately abandon the development of invalid and irrelevant animal models, which may be hampering the progress in research. Importantly, this will result in efforts for the development of good animal models and their validation, which will improve the likelihood that the benefits of research are delivered.

QUESTIONS FOR DISCUSSION AND REFLECTION

1. How shall animal harm in relation to animal research be assessed according to European Directive 2010//63/EU?
2. What are the core elements of each of the 3Rs? Discuss if they sometimes can come into conflict with (a) the scientific goals and (b) each other.
3. What problems may be related to estimating and describing the potential benefits of animal research?
4. What ethically relevant issues are related to translating results from one species to another? What can be done to improve translation?

REFERENCES

APC (Animal Procedures Committee). (2003). Review of Cost-Benefit Assessment in the Use of Animals in Research. Report of the Cost-benefit Working Group of the Animal Procedures Committee. Home Office, Communication Directorate, London.

Button, K.S. Ioannidis, J.P.A. Mokrysz, C. Nosek, B.A. Flint, J. Robinson, E.S.J. & Munafo, M.R. (2013). Power failure: Why small sample size undermines the reliability of neuroscience. *Nature Reviews Neuroscience*, 14: 365–376.

CCAC (Canadian Council on Animal Care). (1991). CCAC policy statement on: categories of invasiveness in animal experiments. http://www.ccac.ca/en_/ standards/policies/policy-categories_of_invasiveness (accessed 12 December 2016).

Duncan, I.J.H. Fraser, D. (1997). Understanding animal welfare. In M.C. Appleby & B.O. Hughes (eds.), *Animal welfare*. Oxfordshire: CABI Publishing.

Dwan, K. Altman, D.G. Arnaiz, J.A. Bloom, J. Chan, A-W. Cronin, E. Decullier, E. Easterbrook, P.J. von Elm, E. Gamble, C. Ghersi, D. Ioannidis, J.P.A. Simes & J. Williamson, P.R. (2008). Systematic review of the empirical evidence of study publication bias and outcome reporting bias. *PLoS ONE*, 3:e3081.

EurActive. (2013). Third successful citizens' petition calls for end to animal testing. http://www.euractiv.com/pa/third-successful-citizens-petiti-news-531404 (accessed 12 December 2016).

European Commission. (2012). Working document on a severity assessment framework. http://ec.europa.eu/environment/chemicals/lab_animals/pdf/Endorsed_Severity_Assessment.pdf (accessed 12 December 2016).

European Commission. (2013a). Examples to illustrate the process of severity classification, day-to-day assessment and actual severity assessment. http:// ec.europa.eu/environment/chemicals/lab_animals/pdf/examples.pdf (accessed January 2017).

European Commission. (2013b). Seventh report on the statistics on the number of animals used for experimental and other scientific purposes in the member states of the European Union. http://eur-lex.europa.eu/legal-content/EN/ TXT/?uri=CELEX:52013DC0859 (accessed 12 December 2016).

Franco, N.H. (2013). Animal experiments in biomedical research: A historical perspective. *Animals*, 3: 238–273.

Franco, N.H. & Olsson, I.A.S. (2012). 'How sick must your mouse be?' – An analysis of the use of animal models in huntington's disease research. *Atla-Alternatives to Laboratory Animals*, 40: 271–283.

Gama Sosa, M. De Gasperi & R. Elder, G. (2012). Modeling human neurodegenerative diseases in transgenic systems. *Human Genetics*, 131: 535–563.

Honess, P. & Wolfensohn, S. (2010). The extended welfare assessment grid: A matrix for the assessment of welfare and cumulative suffering in experimental animals. *Atla-Alternatives to Laboratory Animals*, 38: 205–212.

Ito, R. Takahashi, T. Katano, I. & Ito, M. (2012). Current advances in humanized mouse models. *Cellular & Molecular Immunology*, 9: 208–214.

Katz, D.M. Berger-Sweeney, J.E. Eubanks, J.H. Justice, M.J. Neul, J.L. Pozzo-Miller, L. Blue, M.E. Christian, D. Crawley, J.N. & Giustetto, M. (2012). Preclinical research in Rett syndrome: Setting the foundation for translational success. *Disease Models & Mechanisms*, 5: 733–745.

National Research Council (NRC). (2005). Committee on Applications of Toxicogenomics to Cross-Species Extrapolation. Application of Toxicogenomics to Cross-Species Extrapolation: A Report of a Workshop. Washington DC. National Academies Press (US).

Olsson, I.A.S. (2010). Measuring welfare. In D.S. Mills, J.N. Marchant-Forde, P.D. McGereevy, D.B. Morton, C.J. Nicol, C.J.C. Phillips, P. Sandøe & R.R. Swaisgood (eds.), *Encyclopedia of applied animal behaviour and welfare*. Oxfordshire: CABI Publishing, pp. 407–408.

Olsson, I.A.S. Franco, N.H. Weary, D.M. Sandøe, P. (2011). The 3Rs principle – mind the ethical gap! *ALTEX*, 29: 333–336.

Pound, P. Bracken, M.B. (2014). Is animal research sufficiently evidence based to be a cornerstone of biomedical research? *TheBMJ*, 348.

Richardson, C.A. & Flecknell, P.A. (2005). Anaesthesia and post-operative analgesia following experimental surgery in laboratory rodents: Are we making progress? *Alternatives to Laboratory Animals: ATLA*, 33: 119–127.

Russell, W. & Burch, R. (1959). *The principles of humane experimental technique*. London: Methuen & Co. Ltd.

Sena, E.S. van der Worp, H.B. Bath, P.M.W. Howells, D.W. & Macleod, M.R. (2010). Publication bias in reports of animal stroke studies leads to major overstatement of efficacy. *Plos Biology*, 8: e1000344.

Shultz, L.D. Brehm, M.A. Garcia, J.V. & Greiner, D.L. (2012). Humanized mice for immune system investigation: Progress, promise and challenges. *Nature Reviews Immunology*, 12: 786–798.

Smith, J.A. & Boyd, K.M. (1991). *Lives in the balance: The ethics of using animals in biomedical research*. Oxford: Oxford University Press.

Smith, J.A. van den Broek, F.A.R. Martorell, J.C. Hackbarth, H. Ruksenas, O. & Zeller, W. (2007). Principles and practice in ethical review of animal experiments across Europe: Summary of the report of a FELASA working group on ethical evaluation of animal experiments. *Laboratory Animals*, 41: 143–160.

Spangenberg, E.M. & Keeling, L.J. (2016). Assessing the welfare of laboratory mice in their home environment using animal-based measures – a benchmarking tool. *Laboratory Animals*, 50: 30–38.

U.S. Department of Health and Human Services Food and Drug Administration (FDA). (2014). Product Development Under the Animal Rule: Guidance for Industry.http://www.fda.gov/downloads/drugs/guidancecomplianceregulatory information/guidances/ucm399217.pdf (Accessed 2016-12-12).

van der Worp, H.B. de Haan, P. Morrema, E. & Kalkman, C.J. (2005). Methodological quality of animal studies on neuroprotection in focal cerebral ischaemia. *Journal of Neurology*, 252: 1108–1114.

Varga, O.E. Zsíros, N. & Olsson, I.A. (2015). Estimating the predictive validity of diabetic animal models in rosiglitazone studies. *Obesity Reviews*, 16: 498–507.

WellcomeTrust. (2015). Statement supporting European Directive 2010/63/EU' on the protection of animals used for scientific purposes. https://wellcome .ac.uk/sites/default/files/stop-vivisection-initiative-joint-statement-mar15 .pdf (accessed 12 December 2016).

Wolfensohn, S. Sharpe, S. Hall, I. Lawrence, S. Kitchen, S. & Dennis, M. (2015). Refinement of welfare through development of a quantitative system for assessment of lifetime experience. *Animal Welfare*, 24: 139–149.

World Organization for Animal Health (OIE). (2014). Terrestrial Animal Health Code. 25th Ed. ISBN of volume I: 978-92-95108-01-1 Chapter 7.1, Article 7.1.1. http://www.oie.int/en/international-standard-setting/terrestrial-code/

Yeates, J.W. (2010). Death is a welfare issue. *Journal of Agricultural & Environmental Ethics*, 23: 229–241.

4 Applying Ethical Thinking and Social Relevance

With Franck L.B. Meijboom (Section 4.3)

In the preceding chapters, normative ethical theories, key concepts of research ethics and animal ethics have been presented, including the legislative basis for ethical evaluation (harm–benefit), the 3Rs and relevance of research in terms of translation. In the present chapter, these concepts and theories are applied using concrete examples of animal research. In Section 4.1, a number of recent examples from different research fields are presented, based on which some examples of what ethical issues arise and how an ethical scrutiny can be performed are presented in Section 4.2. Societal aspects and how to take them into account are discussed in Section 4.3.

4.1 RESEARCH ON ANIMALS: EXAMPLES OF DIFFERENT PURPOSES AND IMPACTS

Different research projects result in very different impact on animals, ranging from below the threshold for legislation in many countries (e.g. observational research of animals living in their natural environment) to severe (e.g. inducing severe diseases). As an illustration of different kinds of projects and how to consider the different aspects of their impact on research animals, we here present a list of projects of different severity. In order to ensure that the examples are realistic and up to date, they have been selected from research papers published in 2014–2015.[1] Wildlife, biomedical and agricultural applications are covered in studies carried out in several European countries as well as the United States, Japan and Brazil. An overview of the studies is presented in Table 4.1.

---

[1] A Pubmed search for the term 'disease' with the filter 'other animals' was carried out on 27 April 2015. Abstracts and papers were checked until a sufficient number of examples for each severity category had been found.

Table 4.1 *List of projects on wildlife, biomedical and agricultural applications performed in different countries exemplifying different degrees of severity and different aims in the light of societal relevance.*

Example	What is the social relevance of the study?[a]	What is done to the animals?	What will the animals experience?	Severity
1) Genetic diagnosis in bovine embryos (Kageyama et al., 2015)	If successful, this method will permit breeding for healthy animals without decreasing the gene pool. This is relevant for animal production and gene diversity in a small breed.	Administration of FSH (follicle-stimulating hormone) to cows. Artificial insemination. Flushing through insertion of a catheter into the uterine horn to obtain embryos.	FSH administration leads to superovulation which may be painful Flushing done under regional anaesthesia (epidural). 6–7 day embryos are not covered by legislation and thus severity classification does not apply.	Mild

(continued)

Table 4.1 (continued)

Example	What is the social relevance of the study?[a]	What is done to the animals?	What will the animals experience?	Severity
2) Oral vaccination of wild white-footed mice to prevent Lyme disease transmission (Richer et al., 2014)	This example addresses a disease that is widely recognized as a serious threat to human health and tests a potential strategy for the prevention of Lyme disease transmission.	Live-trap capture of wild white-footed mice Trapped mice are ear tagged, weighed and inspected. Selected mice are brought to the laboratory for blood sampling (100µl).	Stress while kept in the live trap. Maximum time in trap is around 15h. Additional stress from handling. Both restraint and handling stress is increased for mice which are selected for blood sampling. Repeated exposure to stressful procedures (a mouse recaptured on average 6.5 times).	*Moderate*
3) Effect of food emulsifiers on mouse gut microbiota and health (Chassaing et al., 2015)	The aim is to understand the role of widely used food additives in the increase of widespread human health problems.	Exposure to emulsifiers (food additives) through drinking water. Fasting for up to 15 h Gavage	Emulsifier administration leads to colitis in some mice. Stress in particular from gavage which is a particularly aversive administration technique. Accumulated experience per animal not clear from the paper.	*Moderate* for mice which develop colitis, possibly *mild* for the remaining mice unless repeated gavage

Study	Aim	Procedure	Description	Severity
4) Peridontal disease rats (Scarabelot *et al.*, 2014)	The aim is to get scientific knowledge and to understand how exposure to high levels of corticosteroids affects disease development. This could later lead to better treatments.	Ligature placement around second maxillary molar (under general anaesthesia) Corticosteroid inhalation in ventilation chamber.	Ligatures remain in place for 15 days, during which gingival inflammation develops.	Moderate
5) Vaccination in broilers (Dortmans *et al.*, 2014)	Testing the efficacy of vaccinating broiler chickens against Newcastle disease improves animal health and food safety.	Intranasal / intratracheal administration of virulent Newcastle disease virus strains to broiler chickens.	Animals with suboptimal immunity will be infected and develop Newcastle disease. Clinical signs include breathing difficulty, neurological signs, diarrhoea and general sickness. 50–100% of birds (depending on virus strain and bird immune status) died within 14 days after infection.	Severe

(continued)

Table 4.1 *(continued)*

Example	What is the social relevance of the study?[a]	What is done to the animals?	What will the animals experience?	Severity
6) Graft-versus-host disease in mice (Theiss-Suennemann *et al.*, 2015)	The project's direct aim is to test the effect of glucocorticoids on acute graft-versus-host disease. The results could lead to better treatments.	Total body irradiation Intravenous injection with transplanted bone marrow and T-cells or spleen cells.	Transplantation leads to graft-to-host disease (transplanted immune cells attack host tissue with damage of the liver, skin, mucosa and gastrointestinal tract. All animals reached severe graft-to-host disease (at which point they were euthanized) within 45 days after transplantation.	Severe

[a] Social relevance refers not only to human health and welfare but also to effects on animals and nature, as well as overall economic and societal situation. The aspects mentioned in the table are by necessity fewer than those elaborated on in the text.

Source: Original table by Meijboom, Röcklinsberg, Gjerris and Olsson.

In the first example, a genetic analysis is carried out on cattle embryos. The objective is to develop a method to diagnose genetic diseases, to be used in a cattle breed with small genetic diversity and significant problems with hereditary pathologies. The animals involved in the harm analysis here are the donor cows, since 6–7 days post-conception is too early in the developmental stage for the embryos to be considered potentially sentient or to be covered by legislation. The embryo production and collection involves hormonal stimulation to make the cows superovulate (in order to be able to harvest a large number of embryos for each cow), followed by artificial insemination and flushing of the uterus. Stimulation with follicle-stimulating hormone is done through daily injections for 3 days, and the main impact is probably not the injections, but the effects of superovulation, which is potentially painful (van Reenen, 2009). Artificial insemination and embryo harvest both involves inserting a catheter through the cervix, which the technician is locating through inserting their other hand in the rectum of the cow. Artificial insemination takes a couple of minutes and is done without anaesthesia. To harvest the embryos, a catheter is inserted through the vagina into the uterus, and saline solution is slowly flushed through the uterus. The size of a cow allows the procedure to be done non-surgically and with the cow awake and standing, using epidural anaesthesia to anaesthetize the genital region. The process is similar to that used in cattle breeding and does not cause persistent harm to the cow beyond the relatively short-lasting discomfort associated with superovulation and with the flushing procedure. Therefore, the appropriate classification for this experiment seems to be *mild*.

In the second example, wild-living white-footed mice are studied to evaluate how effective an oral vaccine is in preventing Lyme disease infection. The objective is to explore ways to reduce human exposure by vaccinating the wild reservoir host. White-footed mice are caught using baited live traps. The bait is also the vehicle for the oral vaccine. Traps are set up late in the afternoon and checked approximately 15 hours later. Mice which are caught are equipped with an individual ear tag, weighed and inspected and released again. In addition, randomly selected mice are brought to the laboratory for a blood sample to be taken. Impact on the animals in this experiment is above all stress from capture and handling of these wild animals with no experience of human contact. In the case of mice which are captured, ear tagged and inspected, this stress is classified as mild, since human contact is very brief and the period which the animals are kept in the trap is minimized to that necessary to ensure that enough mice are indeed trapped, i.e. covering the dark period of the day when these nocturnal animals are active. Blood sampling subjects the mice to a longer period in captivity (not specified in the paper), more extensive manipulation and transport. On average, each mouse was captured 6.5 times and blood-sampled once. Even though there is minimal physical intervention with the animals, the stress reaction likely to be evoked in wild mice trapped for up to 15 hours justifies a classification as *moderate* rather than *mild*.

In the third example, laboratory mice are used to study how food emulsifiers affect gut microbiota and metabolic health. The objective is to understand the potential role of dietary emulsifier in inflammatory bowel disease and metabolic syndrome. Mice are administered different food emulsifiers through their drinking water for three months, and thereafter different parameters are measured. At the end of treatment, blood is collected through the retroorbital approach, immediately followed by euthanasia and organ collection. Other parameter measurements imply different combinations of fasting (4–15 hours) and substance administration through gavage. It is not clear how the procedures are combined in individual mice. Some mice develop colitis as an effect of the emulsifier treatment. The retroorbital blood sampling method is controversial, but the main problem (post-sampling complications if not correctly executed) does not apply in this experiment, as the mice are euthanized immediately after blood sampling. However, it may be possible to change the order so that blood is drawn immediately after euthanasia. The impact of fasting depends on the duration, and the longest fasting here is overnight (15 hours), which is within the mild range according to Directive 2010/63/EU. Gavage may be aversive but, if done by a skilled technician, mice are likely to habituate to the procedure, which is short lasting. Colitis (inflammation of the colon) is an unintended side effect affecting some of the mice. Considering that individual mice may experience several of the procedures as well as the pathology, the study should be classified as *moderate* even though for some mice it may be *mild*.

In the fourth example, periodontal disease is induced in laboratory rat in order to understand how exposure to high levels of corticosteroids affects disease development. To induce periodontal inflammation, cotton ligatures are placed around one of the molars (procedure is performed under general anaesthesia). Corticosteroids are administered in a forced ventilation chamber where the animals inhale the nebulized drug once per day. After 15 days, the animals are euthanized and all measures are taken post-mortem. The study implies induction of a disease which is painful. Although the pain is localized to a small area, the mouth and teeth are particularly sensitive areas, and it therefore seems most appropriate to classify the study as *moderate*.

In the fifth example, the efficacy of vaccinating broiler chickens against Newcastle disease is studied (Figure 4.1). Chickens are obtained from farms, where they had either been vaccinated under field conditions (oral vaccine in drinking water) or not vaccinated. In addition, a group of non-vaccinated SPF (specific pathogen free) chickens from the same farm is included. All animals are intranasally/intratracheally exposed to Newcastle disease virus of different strains. Unless the vaccine confers effective protection, this virus challenge will cause birds to develop Newcastle disease, which in unprotected birds progressively lead to death. After the challenge, the animals are observed daily for 14 days or until found dead, whatever happens first. Survival varies between groups, but at least 50% of birds die from Newcastle disease, with 100% mortality in the non-vaccinated SPF group. Since the study implies full disease development leading up to death for a proportion of the animals, the appropriate classification is *severe*.

In the sixth example, the effect of glucocorticoids on acute graft-versus-host disease is tested in laboratory mice. To knock out the immune system, mice are exposed to total body radiation. Subsequently, bone marrow and T-cells or spleen cells from mice of a different genetic background are transplanted through intravenous injection. This transplantation leads to the development of acute graft-versus-host disease, in which the transplanted immune cells attack the host tissue which is perceived as foreign, since the host and the immune cell donor are genetically different. All animals developed severe graft-versus-host disease and reached the predefined humane endpoint (losing 20% body weight or moribund) state within 45 days after transplantation. Since the study implies full disease development leading up to death (euthanasia of moribund animals), the appropriate classification is *severe*.

4.2 RESEARCH ON ANIMALS IN THE LIGHT OF DIFFERENT ETHICAL THEORIES

In this section we will discuss the preceding examples as seen from the perspectives of the ethical theories presented in Chapter 2. This will show how a certain research protocol – or any ethically loaded situation, for that matter – is perceived differently depending on the ethical position from which it is evaluated.

From a *contractarian* point of view, the only considerations to take is how using the animals in these different ways will affect the evaluator. Will s/he in the long run be better able to obtain her goals by doing it? Or would s/he be better off by taking a stance against some or all of the experiments? How does the use of animals in research affect the social contracts that s/he has entered? The calculations of the economic or social effects of different positions might be complicated, but at no point in the equation are any of the animals regarded as anything but a mean to achieve the researcher's ends. Such an ethical position can be regarded as rather extreme, and since it does not consider animal welfare at all, it is not relevant for further consideration here. Please note that this is not a dismissal of the philosophical qualities of the position, but a pragmatic choice based on the fact that most legislation on animal research grant animals some protection. This is explicit in Recital 12 of the EU directive (2010/63/EU), which implicitly dismisses the position by stating that animals have an intrinsic value that must be respected and that concerns of the general public are relevant:

> Animals have an intrinsic value which must be respected. There are also the ethical concerns of the general public as regards the use of animals in procedures. Therefore, animals should always be treated as sentient creatures and their use in procedures should be restricted to areas which may ultimately benefit human or animal health, or the environment.

Someone holding an *animal rights* view could, contrary to values implicit in most legislation on research animals, argue that in example 1 (genetic analysis on cattle embryos) the cow that is impregnated with the calf can be seen as a victim of instrumentalization. Independently of the level of welfare impairment, she is wrongly used as a tool to produce embryos, rather than respected in herself. Further, the embryos are also harmed. Even though they are not caused suffering, they may still be wronged due to their reduction to an instrument for human purposes. A similar critique would apply in example 5 (Newcastle disease in chickens), where the entire purpose of the study would be questioned. Departing from the position that each animal is subject in its own life, large-scale poultry production is unacceptable from the outset. Inducing a disease which we know causes the birds to suffer in order to study a vaccine that will enable such production systems cannot be justified. On the other hand, since Newcastle disease spread also in free range or extensive housed chickens, this is a welfare issue independent of housing system. However, development of the vaccine is probably motivated by economic interests also associated with the high-intensity production systems, something not approved by an animal rights defender. An animal rights position on example 3 (wild mouse) is not necessarily as critical. Even though the capture and blood sampling is unpleasant for the mice, the vaccine will improve their health, and hence could be regarded as less of an instrumentalization. There are many discussions within the animal rights community as to what human obligations towards wild animals are: leaving them alone or interfering to improve their lives? That is, unlike when developing a vaccine which may improve the health of animals which the animal rightist thinks should not be kept anyway (chickens for meat or egg production), the health gain for wild mice might be accepted from the animal right's point of view.

On the other hand, if animal rights prevailed, there would be much fewer chickens around, which from a *utilitarian* position could be an issue if one takes the goal of maximization of utility (e.g. happiness or preferences) seriously. If, all things considered, chickens in this study have a good enough life to add preference satisfaction to the total 'account', then they should be bred. Given the classification of 'severe' in the description above, this is, however, most probably not the case and shows that animal welfare assessment would be a central part from a utilitarian position, contrary to an animal rights position. From the latter, however, if a study also includes genetic modification, the question of whether or not this is acceptable as such is evoked. A rights position may describe this as an additional harm to the individual animal by its obvious instrumentalization, besides the harm caused by the effects of the modification and the experiment.

In general, the utilitarian position finds that the amount of welfare lost and won through the actual experiment on the animals needs to be weighed against the possible costs and gains that will come out of it. Factors that should be taken into account are the economic costs and possible gains, the effect on all involved – from animal caretakers, to people benefitting from the results, to people experiencing a welfare loss because of their objection to animal experimentation. The pain and suffering of the mice in example 6 is thus justifiable as long as the potential benefits are realistic and large enough to outweigh them. In general there is nothing wrong with using sentient individuals for research as long as the welfare of all welfare-capable beings affected by the research is maximized. It will therefore depend on a case-by-case analysis that, as discussed in Chapter 2, often will rest on guesstimates of the positive and negative effects of the research. It is therefore necessary to gain as much information as possible and be very open about the assumptions underlying the evaluation of e.g. the importance of the welfare loss of the animals to make a valuable utilitarian analysis of a specific case.

Example 2 and parts of 3 (wild-living white-footed mice and food emulsifiers and euthanasia at 3 months) are rather uncomplicated from a *utilitarian* position. Although undoubtedly stressful for the wild mice to be caught or have blood sampled from behind the eye, the suffering is relatively limited, and given that the chance of a positive outcome of the study is high, the benefits will typically be evaluated to outweigh the harms. In example 3 the mice are euthanized and that should, from the utilitarian standpoint, ideally be compensated by bringing other beings into life, with comparable or better welfare, or by increasing the overall welfare in other ways in order to be acceptable. From both *virtue* and *feminist care ethical positions*, the wild mouse example is more interesting, though. What kind of researcher am I, to catch and stress innocent wild mice? On the other hand, it might be the only defendable way to get hold of research animals, as they are not bred and caged for their entire life, and are also released again. Could it be that the fact that I vaccinate them (i.e. boost their health) compensates for the welfare impairment through ear tagging and blood sampling? Is this to embody the virtue of kindness or the vice of putting other's interests aside to obtain my own goals? From a *care ethics* perspective, it is relevant to focus on the possibility to take care of non-domesticated mice. Compared to mice used to human handling, caging, indoor smells and sounds etc. – everything is frightening, and even the gentlest handling possible

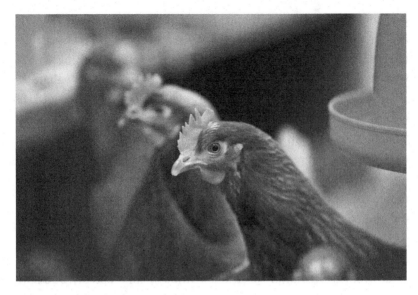

FIGURE 4.1 Brown hens.

Source: Image © Understanding Animal Research, www.understandinganimalresearch .org.uk.

comes foreign to them. Hence, what is relevant to ensure according to feminist ethics of care cannot be ensured, and therefore makes the study difficult to approve.

From both a *virtue ethics* position and according to *feminist ethics or ethics of care*, studies as in examples 4 (periodontal disease), 5 (Newcastle disease) and 6 (the effect of glucocorticoids on acute graft-versus-host disease) are difficult to approve. In these examples the induction of disease and drug administration/vaccine treatment causing pain and the killing in itself might be contrary to how a caring person is considering him/herself. Although consequences should be taken into consideration in discernment of a situation, neither virtue ethics nor feminist ethics regards a comparison of outcomes and harms to be a sufficient approach, hence potentially high benefits cannot in themselves be a carte blanche to proceed. These positions rather ask if the individual needs of the animals are met, how it is housed and fed etc. In none of these cases the needs and preferences of the animals are met, and in case 6 animals are even kept alive until a late endpoint, and individual needs are severely harmed. A person holding a virtue ethics position would also ask if this kind of handling of animals is compatible with the ideals of being a wise, just and attentive person. Attention to human needs is important, and open for use of animals, but also attention to animal needs is crucial.

It is also relevant to consider the need for the potential benefit, i.e. need of the resulting information also for both virtue and feminist care ethicists. This is perhaps easier to evaluate in example 5, possibly coming to the conclusion that a new vaccine against Newcastle Disease is not necessary, as the entire standard housing of chickens is contrary to what a virtue ethicist and feminist care ethicist would accept. Regarding example 4 and 6, the expected benefits are not as clearly expressed, and perhaps difficult to evaluate, but as the level of animal harm is high, i.e. total lack of individual care and attention, acceptability from a virtue or feminist ethics is not probable.

As shown here, the different ethical perspectives will evaluate the cases differently. This is worth keeping in mind when one enters ethical discussions on animal research in general or on specific cases. The reasons for disagreements are hence not necessarily based on lack of knowledge from some of the participants or their unwillingness to listen to common sense. Often it is based on different value perspectives. Also, outside academic philosophy, we rarely see pure utilitarianism, pure virtue ethics etc; what we see is that elements of the different theories often appear in any discussion of an ethically challenging situation. Against this background, discussing ethically laden issues against these positions might not lead to a shared agreement, but it could lead to a higher degree of understanding and respect for those that do not share the same opinions – and thus in the end lead to more socially robust compromises on how to proceed with animal research.

4.3 SEARCHING FOR SOCIAL RELEVANCE: COMPLEX EVALUATION OF ANIMAL RESEARCH

In the previous section different types of research were discussed, demonstrating a variety in classification of harm. This harm assessment, however, is only one part of the ethical evaluation of animal-based research. It is also a matter of benefits. Researchers aim to achieve certain goals by doing animal research. In some cases the research goal lies exclusively on scientific progress, but quite often a social relevance is claimed, and hence this social significance has to be included in the ethical assessment of a research project. However, legal documents and professional guidelines often lack clear and practical guidance with regard to the assessment of the relevance and benefit of an experiment (Grimm, 2014; Vieira de Castro and Olsson, 2015). This is not the result of indifference, but an indication that the evaluation of the (social) relevance of animal research is not an easy task. This section aims to get a grip on the social relevance of animal research. What is the social significance of a specific research project and can it be distinguished from scientific aims? Why is the evaluation of social relevance difficult in real life, and is it possible to deal with this complexity? These questions are discussed in what follows.

4.3.1 *When Does an Aim Have Social Relevance?*

If one discusses with researchers why they use animals for research, there often is no single answer. For instance, in the case of the animal experiment in which periodontal disease is induced in laboratory rats (see Section 4.1), the aim is increased scientific knowledge, but the context and final aim of this research is to understand how exposure to high levels of corticosteroids affects disease development. The latter is also of social relevance because it can contribute to improved treatments and lead to a better health status of humans. This shows that there often is not a clear watershed between the scientific and the social relevance of use of animals in research. One can even stress that science is of public importance too and thus has social relevance.

Nonetheless, the EU-directive and the compulsory ethical assessments of animal research use the distinction between the scientific and the social relevance. This does not deny that research as such can be socially relevant, but it stresses that animal research can contribute to other public goods and therefore have social relevance. This is important because it entails that the evaluation of the relevance of a specific animal test is beyond the (global) research community. It requires public participation.

Research projects aiming to contribute to social and moral values, such as human health and safety, animal welfare or environmental safety are said to be of social relevance. It might be indirect by requiring time and efforts in several steps. For example, the development of genetic diagnosis of bovine embryos (case 1) can contribute to protection of traditional breeds by minimizing the risk of inbreeding. In other cases, innovations might lead to more efficient handling of nature resources and public goods opening for economic redistribution in the public sector. Actually, all research projects presented in Section 4.1 claim social relevance in either the short or the long run. For instance, the project that aims to test the effect of glucocorticoids on acute graft-versus-host disease is linked to the value of human health. Similarly, the project that focuses on the efficacy of vaccinating broiler chickens against Newcastle disease claims social relevance as it is linked to animal health and food safety. However, a relevant aim alone is not sufficient basis for an ethical justification; the likelihood to achieve the aim and the animal suffering required to do so also need to be considered.

4.3.2 *Problems of Probability and Uncertainty*

In order to make an ethical assessment, we need to evaluate the societal relevance of the project. That, however, is easier said than done. A first hurdle has to do with problems of probability and uncertainty. Research with animals is evaluated before the actual experiment takes place. Therefore, one can never be completely certain about whether the direct or final aim will be reached. There is always an element of uncertainty and probability. Suppose we would agree that a certain aim is of high social relevance, for instance a method that prevents the development of amyotrophic lateral sclerosis (ALS). Then the ethical assessment of the animal use still requires an assessment of the probability that this aim will be reached by the envisaged steps taken in a project. Therefore, one can have serious objections against an experiment with a clear social significance if there is a low probability that this aim is actually reached, e.g. given the choice of the research design.

This picture is further complicated by the fact that one project can have various aims. The research examples presented in Section 4.1 have clear goals, but if one takes a closer look, it is possible to discern various aims in each of the examples. For instance, in the case of the project on Newcastle disease, the aim is primarily on animal health, but also includes aims linked to improving the level of food production. Vaccine development aims to improve animal health, which in turn may reduce the risk for transmission of zoonotic diseases from animals to humans, and in the case of bacterial infections (Newcastle disease is caused by a virus) also reduction of the use of antibiotics in animal production. Therefore, it is necessary to take the relevance and the probability of all the aims of a project into account. For instance, if researchers indicate that they aim to contribute to the development of improved therapeutics for colon cancer, it is likely that the aim will be assessed as very relevant. However, given the scientific and practical complexity related to drug development, it remains uncertain whether they will succeed, even if the researchers have well-defined hypotheses and perform their experiments carefully. The chance that they reach their additional aim, e.g. to validate their newly established animal model, is much more likely. However, notwithstanding the relevance of good animal models, it scores lower on societal significance because it has mainly instrumental value that is related to the value of knowledge. This example shows that although it is possible to judge the benefit of research, the interplay between probability and relevance makes it quite difficult to come to clear statements.

4.3.3   *Assessing Social Relevance: Where to Start?*

Now it is possible to move to the question of how to assess the social relevance of a project. To answer that question we first have to deal with the question of where the discussion on social relevance of an animal research project should start. In a discussion of the social relevance of animal research, one is often confronted with different opinions. One reason for this is that the question of the relevance of a project can be discussed on many levels. To get a better grip on these discussions, it helps to differentiate between three related levels:

(a)   the societal context or background of the animal research;
(b)   the final aim of the animal experiment;
(c)   the direct aim of the animal experiment.

Concerning (a), animal research often starts in a specific societal context such as the increased incidence of obesity-related health problems or the role aquaculture can play in securing food security. This, for instance, is the reason why a project gets funding or media attention. At this level the relation between public moral values and ethical principles often is relatively clear. However, in most cases the problems at stake appear to be too complex to be solved by one research project. If we take again the example of vaccinating broiler chickens against Newcastle disease, one could introduce this project as part of the wider development towards sustainable food production. This latter ambition will probably be considered by many as an important and valuable aim. Nonetheless, a mere reference to this overall aim will not suffice to judge the social significance of a project on the efficacy of vaccinating chickens. It only works if the relation between striving for sustainable food production and the specific project can been explicated. However, this is not an easy task. On the one hand, to indicate how vaccinating animals contributes to sustainability is difficult in empirical terms, because both immunology and sustainability are highly complex fields. On the other hand, the plurality of definitions of sustainability, views on the role animal production can play and ideas about animal health indicate that there is more than an empirical challenge: there is an ethical problem. The discussion is about values and value conflicts. For instance, the researcher may stress that his project clearly has social relevance because of the importance of healthy animals for sustainable food production, while someone else stresses that the social relevance of this project on vaccination is rather limited because it still starts in the current poultry industry and overlooks the need of a more fundamental change to sustainable food production. Such differences or conflicts cannot be easily solved in the context of animal research. They are better addressed at the level of public debate, science policy or politics. For this context, it is important to note that one has to be careful when referring to broad societal challenges in order to stress the social significance of a specific project.

This leads to the second level, (b), at which the social relevance of a project can be discussed. This focuses on the final aim of the project. In our case, one could define this in terms of the aim to develop a vaccine that confers effective protection and therefore to prevent poultry from dying due to the disease. This, however, suggests two aims: less incidence of Newcastle disease and the market introduction of new vaccines. It is obvious that at this level the relation between the aim and the specific project is much stronger than on the previous level. However, there still are uncertainties at this stage. For instance, if the final aim is market introduction of new vaccines, the question whether this aim will be reached does not only depend on the success of this animal research. It requires more research, a long registration process with the authorities and dealing with market circumstances. For the debate on the social relevance it also touches upon issue of the double aim. Most of us will value healthy animals, and if vaccines can contribute to that value, this appears useful. However, we already have vaccines for chicken available. This raises the question: what is the added value of another vaccine? Does it really contribute to the health of the animal or is it more a matter of product development? In practice these questions do not have an easy answer, because it often is not an either-or issue. However, reflection on this question is very important because it is of direct influence on the assessment of an animal research project.

Finally, regarding (c), some argue that the best way to address the discussion on the relevance of an animal experiment is to start with the direct aim of the research. In our case it is the aim to study the efficacy of vaccinating chickens against Newcastle disease. This focus provides us with a better grip on the question about the definition and the feasibility of the aim. If the experiment is well described, it is easy to define what the researcher will do with chickens and why. However, to assess the answer to the question of why, we have to return to other levels. When considering the social relevance of animal-based research, the efficacy of a vaccine cannot be separated from broader questions, such as: 'Why are vaccines important?', 'Why do we need more vaccines?' or 'Why should we have chickens for food production?'

The discussion of the three levels shows the complexity of the assessment of the social relevance. This, however, should not lead to the conclusion that it is impossible to assess this part of the benefit of animal research. It only shows that it requires careful reflection of the answers, and awareness of the level at which one discusses the relevance of a project.

4.3.4 *How to Value the Societal Relevance?*

As a final step, we need to discuss the question of how to value the societal relevance. An obvious answer would be that social relevance is the same as what the society or members of the public consider important. To a certain extent, public opinion is indeed an important parameter. Nonetheless, there is more to say. First, a lot of research projects focus on topics where we lack a clear public opinion. This can be the result of the novel character of the research, for instance in the case of studies that may lead to new treatment for a recently discovered disease. It also can be because of a genuine plurality in society, for instance with regard to the use of gene technology. In these cases it is not (yet) possible to rely on the public opinion.

Second, there are ethical reasons why one should take a broader perspective on social relevance than a mere reference to what the public considers to be important. In ethics, impartiality, consistency and coherency are considered to be indicators of quality. This implies that one takes a perspective that includes the interests of other parties into account, that one addresses and assesses equal cases equally, and that one has a view how one's assessments relate to each other. In practice this implies that it is important to indicate who can potentially benefit. The potential beneficiaries should be conceived in a broad sense, including individual human persons, society, individual animals, animal species, nature and the environment.

Third, it is relevant to explore the ethical values at stake. They have many sources and mirror different focus points in a society. Examples include universal rights such as justice or righteousness, which matter in e.g. decisions on how to distribute research funding; utility or maximization of common good, which is relevant in relation to e.g. research objectives; perfectionist ends of self-development which may influence work environment and publication strategies; and, of course, individual projects to which one is committed (Nagel, 2012). Acknowledging this background makes the argumentation less susceptible to arbitrariness, because it is possible to explain and support why certain values are important.

Finally, the reference to potential beneficiaries and values helps to trace potential conflicts. In the case study of the efficacy of vaccinating chickens such conflicts may occur between the value of economy and animal health, or between the interests of the farmer and those of the pharmaceutical company.

These three steps will not result in objective outcomes, but they enable to understand nuances in different perceptions, explain and support one's view on the social relevance of an animal research project and make a dialogue possible. These are essential steps in the assessment of the social relevance of an animal experiment and for the broader question of the ethical assessment of animal research in general.

QUESTIONS FOR DISCUSSION AND REFLECTION

1. Describe your own research, or animal-based research that you are part of or know well, using the same structure as used for the six examples given in this chapter, summarized in Table 4.1. This description will be the basis for the questions that follow.
2. How would the different ethical theories evaluate that research? What aspects are of core relevance in each of the theories?
3. Describe and reflect upon the potential benefits that could grow out of that research and compare them to the potential harm and welfare loss experienced by the animal.
4. What values should govern the understanding of what is 'socially relevant' in that research? Are there other socially relevant values?

REFERENCES

Chassaing, B. Koren, O. Goodrich, J.K. Poole, A.C. Srinivasan, S. Ley, R.E. & Gewirtz, A.T. (2015). Dietary emulsifiers impact the mouse gut microbiota promoting colitis and metabolic syndrome. *Nature*, 519: 92–96.

Dortmans, J.C.F.M. Venema-Kemper, S. Peeters, B.P.H. & Koch, G. (2014). Field vaccinated chickens with low antibody titres show equally insufficient protection against matching and non-matching genotypes of virulent Newcastle disease virus. *Veterinary Microbiology*, 172: 100–107.

Grimm, H. (2014). Ethics in laboratory animal science. In E. Jensen-Jarolim (ed.), *Comparative medicine* (pp. 281–230). Wien: Springer.

Kageyama, S. Hirayama, H. Moriyasu, S. & Minamihashi, A. (2015). Genetic diagnosis of band 3 deficiency using a quenching probe (QProbe)-PCR assay in bovine embryos. *Japanese Journal of Veterinary Research*, 63: 45–51.

Nagel, T. (2012). *Mortal questions*. Cambridge: Cambridge University Press.

Richer, L.M. Brisson, D. Melo, R. Ostfeld, R.S. Zeidner, N. & Gomes-Solecki, M. (2014). Reservoir targeted vaccine against borrelia burgdorferi: A new strategy to prevent lyme disease transmission. *Journal of Infectious Diseases*, 209: 1972–1980.

Scarabelot, V.L. Cavagni, J. Medeiros, L.F. Detânico, B. Rozisky, J.R. de Souza, A. Daudt, L.D. Gaio, E.J. Ferreira, M.B.C. Rösing, C.K. Battastini, A.M.O. & Torres, I.L.S. (2014). Periodontal disease and high doses of inhaled corticosteroids alter NTPDase activity in the blood serum of rats. *Archives of Oral Biology,* 59: 841–847.

Theiss-Suennemann, J. Jörß, K. Messmann, J.J. Reichardt, S.D. Montes-Cobos, E. Lühder, F. Tuckermann, J.P. Awolff, H. Dressel, R. Gröne, H-J. Strauß, G. & Reichardt, H.M. (2015). Glucocorticoids attenuate acute graft-versus-host disease by suppressing the cytotoxic capacity of CD8+ T cells. *The Journal of Pathology,* 235: 646–655.

van Reenen, C.G. (2009). Assessing the welfare of transgenic farm animals. In M. Engelhard, K. Hagen & M. Boysen (eds.), *Genetic engineering in livestock. New applications and interdisciplinary perspectives. Ethics of science and technology assessment, vol 34.* (pp. 119–143). Berlin: Springer-Verlag.

Vieira de Castro, A.C. Olsson, I.A. (2015). Does the goal justify the methods? Harm and benefit in neuroscience research using animals. *Current topics in behavioral neurosciences,* 19: 47–78.

5 Regulation and Legislation: Overview and Background

With Katarina Cvek (Subsection 5.2.2);
Orsolya E. Varga (Subsection 5.2.3);
Catherine Schuppli and Elisabeth Ormandy
(Section 5.3); Javier Guillén (Section 5.4); and
Franz Gruber (Subsection 5.5.1) and Joana
Fernandes (Subsection 5.5.2)

Use of animals for research purposes has a long history, and criticism and movements to stop animal experimentation have been intensifying since about the nineteenth century. Such criticism has come both from inside the academic community and through public concern. The call for external control has led to the development of regulations and legislation in many parts of the world (Vasbinder *et al.*, 2014). Whereas legislation, ethics review and project authorization processes aim in different ways to promote the 3Rs principle, scientists are ultimately responsible for how research is designed and carried out, and self-regulation within the scientific community is increasingly important. In order to put the current situation into perspective, we start this chapter with a short historical overview of the development of animal experimentation legislation in Section 5.1. In Section 5.2 we describe the development of the current EU Directive 2010/63/EU and summarize its core elements and illuminate the ethical review system. Section 5.3 focuses on the ethical review system in North America, and the systems in Asia, Oceania and Latin America are described in Section 5.4. Finally, Section 5.5 highlights researcher incentives to formulate and implement ethical guidelines.

5.1 HISTORICAL OVERVIEW: DEVELOPMENT OF ANIMAL RESEARCH LEGISLATION

In this section we briefly illuminate the development of animal research to place contemporary European regulation into perspective. The use of animals in research is of course much older than attempts to regulate it are, but intellectual interest in protecting animals probably goes as far back in history as some of the first known studies with animals. For example, during the third century BC, the physicians Herophilus and Erisistratus in Alexandria studied the function of different nerves, and during the second century AD, Galen of Pergamum described these experiments, conducted his own and described methods and instruments for future research. In parallel, writings from ancient Greek philosophers show reasoning in favour of respect for individual animals and against causing harm or suffering (Walters and Portmess, 1999). Hence, different views on animals in respect to human-animal relationship flourished during this period, but there is little doubt the idea of the humans' right to use animals was the dominant one.

Research has probably continuously been performed, but little has been documented or saved for following generations. The rediscovery of Galen's documents during the sixteenth century, however, led to an increased interest in anatomy throughout Europe, which initiated further studies in comparative physiology. Vivisections on animals were performed as public demonstrations without any use of anaesthetics, which did not become available until the mid-nineteenth century (Monamy, 2009). There was no legislation limiting scope or procedures. Although some physicians (researchers) were concerned about the impaired welfare and suffering of the animals, they also argued that increased knowledge was valued higher than respect for animal pain. Others, such as René Descartes (1595–1650), were convinced that non-human animals – lacking reason, free will and soul – could not suffer, and hence could not be caused harm. Rather, animals could be understood as machines, although complex ones, well suited for vivisections.

Some of Descartes' colleagues, and his family, were not convinced by this argument, however, leading to a public discussion of animal capacities and human responsibilities towards them (Preece, 2002, p. 111 ff), which can be seen as an embryo of the anti-vivisection movement – a movement parallel to anti-slavery and early emancipation in its drive for liberation of oppressed groups. Anti-vivisectionism grew in importance in Europe from the nineteenth century onwards, and turned to a more widespread concern in the next century and directly influenced legislation in some countries. Especially in Britain, a vivid debate paved the way for a humanitarian reform movement which already in the eighteenth century led to a generally accepted Christian-inspired doctrine to treat all God's creatures in a decent way. Combined with a growing interest in the utilitarian way of reasoning, animals were gradually included as objects of moral concern (Alexius Borgström, 2009; Mendelsohn, 1987). The first European legislation against cruelty towards animals was the British/English Martins Act from 1822. Half a century later, in 1876, a new, stricter legislation regarding research on animals with more of a *preventive* aim, An Act to amend the Law relating to Cruelty to Animals Act, came into force, by which a number of restrictions on animal research were introduced: painful experiments were acceptable only if new knowledge was gained, if human lives could be saved or human pain relieved; licenses became necessary for performing experiments in education, as well as for all painful experiments; if possible with regard to expected results, the animals should be killed after painful experiments; and researchers should use small animals if possible instead of horses, donkeys, mules, cats and dogs (Alexius Borgström, 2009). In spite of the intention to limit painful experiments through preventive control, the effect was rather on the formal and bureaucratic side, creating rules for its practice, since licenses and actual control were performed by researchers themselves without much public control and involvement (Mendelsohn, 1987).

Establishment of legislation is a slow process, but other countries followed Britain. Germany's federal legislation on animal welfare came in 1871. In the Netherlands abuse was prohibited in the Dutch Penal Code in 1886, whereas animals were protected from public cruelty in the French legislation from 1850. Sweden had its first preventive animal welfare legislation as late as 1944, following a lengthy and heated debate on both vivisections, how much insight the public should have in research, and whether the public had a right to have an opinion on research which began in the 1880s.

It is noteworthy that arguments presented in the early discussions against animal experimentation differ from today's by drawing not primarily on empathy and sentience, but on doubts about the scientific relevance and accuracy of comparing humans and animals. Based on the conviction, prevalent until after establishment of a Darwinian worldview, of a fundamental difference between humans and other animals, it was further considered a heresy to compare humans with any other species and hence to extrapolate knowledge about anatomy and physiology from animals to humans. Why study animals and compare with humans, given such a difference? Anti-vivisectionists later based their argumentation on a principle of justice towards animals. The following British debate built on utilitarianism and on the inclusion of animals in the sphere of objects contributing to the sum of happiness or unhappiness in the world. The continental argumentation rather referred to the idea of human duty to respect the inherent value of individual animals. Further, all of these lines of thought recognize animals as sentient, and argue that humans should show empathy with their capacity to experience pain and suffering. It is noteworthy that today's theological arguments focus on empathy and respect for animals stressing both the common origin in creation and similarities in physiology (Linzay, 1995).

Early arguments supporting animal experimentation, on the other hand, were very similar to today's arguments in stressing the necessity of freedom of research and the value of increased medical knowledge. The general scientific validity of animal-based research has been called into question in the later years, but often the scientific interpretation of an experiment and the assessment of necessary or best method do not seem to be questioned, given that an experiment is argued to be of importance (Olsson *et al.*, 2008; Persson, 2009; Schuppli *et al.*, 2004).

Another element of legislation concerns public insight and control. Historically, arguments contra public control followed the same pattern of argumentation as pro–animal experimentation, i.e. with reference to trust in scientists' discernment and that public control would lack relevance as only scientists can assess welfare and judge what is necessary. Arguments in favour of public control were based on an idea of a 'self-evident' Christian duty to consider animal suffering as morally relevant, trusting that scientists in general share this view (and therefore would have nothing to lose if controlled). This view could be combined with either pro– or anti–animal experimentation (Alexius Borgström, 2009). As the theological basis of moral argumentation has faded away, another alternative has turned out to be the prevalent one – pro-experiment and pro-control – and the British 1876 legislation partly emanated from public opposition and pressure of scientists' public accountability (Monamy, 2009).

In sum, one can see that historically the main public controversy over research with animals has been about the pain and distress caused by experiments, and this remains the predominant ethical issue in animal research. However, the arguments for taking this into consideration have changed over time.

5.2 REGULATION AND REVIEW OF ANIMAL EXPERIMENTS IN THE EU

5.2.1 *Revision of European Legislation Protecting Animals Used in Experiments*

Directive 86/609/EEC regarding the protection of animals used for experimental and other scientific purposes was one of the first European Directives to set standards for animal protection. It was, however, comparatively limited in scope, and by the time the revision process was initiated in 2002, the Directive was widely considered to be outdated and no longer efficient in setting the desired high and harmonized standards for the European research area. A major problem was the great discrepancies between member states, ranging from a mere transposition of the Directive at a very basic level to extensive and potentially more restrictive national legislation.

The European Commission initiated the revision process by establishing a Technical Expert Working Group (TEWG), in which national authorities as well as stakeholder organizations were represented. The TEWG task was to provide scientific/technical advice in response to questions listed in a Commission Thought Starter document. The response was published in 2003 in final reports of the four respective subgroups on (1) scope, (2) authorization, (3) ethical review and (4) cost-benefit analysis. The Commission further sought the opinion of the Animal Health and Welfare Panel of the European Food Safety Authority in regard to animal sentience, origin of experimental animals and euthanasia methods. The TEWG work was followed by a period of internal Commission consultation and drafting leading up to the presentation of the first-draft proposal in the autumn of 2008 (European Commission, 2015).

The revision process was followed closely by the scientific community and NGOs, and also attracted considerable interest from international observers, given that the European Union, along with the European Research Area, is an important player internationally and accounts for a considerable proportion of the biomedical research and animal use in experiments in the world. During the revision period, hearings were organized and policy briefings and statements published by a number of organizations.

The first public draft version of the revised Directive was met with considerable criticism by the research community which feared limitations to research that they considered were unjustified and which they argued would interfere with the possibilities for scientists and industry to operate within the European Research Area (Anonymous, 2008; FELASA, 2007). This debate was coupled with intense political battle over the new Directive in the European Institutions (European Parliament Legislative Observatory, 2010).

The turbulent process leading up to the finally accepted Directive agreed upon by the European Commission, the European Parliament and the European Council on 7 April 2010 was aptly described by the scientific journal *Nature* as 'more than a decade of pitched battles between research advocates and animal-rights campaigners' (Abbott, 2010).

Directive 2010/63/EU introduces substantial changes compared to 86/609/EEC. It aims to protect animal welfare as a value of the EU and to eliminate disparities in legislation and practice between member states. Important new features include extended scope, enhanced focus on the 3Rs and alternative methods, mandatory project evaluation, severity classification and retrospective assessment, as well as revised guidelines for accommodation and care, which are now mandatory. EU Directives must be transposed into national legislation, and thus the way that the Directive is interpreted nationally will have implications for its practical impact. The implementation of 2010/63/EU is being carefully monitored by the Commission, through meetings with national contact points generating consensus documents for a common interpretation and implementation of the Directive, and Expert Working Groups working at a more technical level to implement sections of the Directive.

5.2.2 *Directive 2010/63/EU in Summary*

The scope of the Directive is to harmonize the legislation protecting the animals used in scientific procedures within the EU as well as making it more stringent and transparent. The main incitement for revising this legislation was the need to improve the welfare of these animals. This was actualized by the increasing scientific knowledge of factors that influence animal welfare, and the capacity of animals to sense and express pain and suffering as well as the ethical concerns of the general public. According to the Lisbon treaty of the functioning of the European Union, Article 13 (Part One, Title II), full regard must be paid to the welfare requirements of animals since they are sentient beings. It was recognized that animals have an intrinsic value which must be respected and that animals should always be treated as sentient creatures and their use in procedures should be restricted to areas which may ultimately benefit human or animal health, or the environment. An overarching aim of the Directive is to replace, refine and reduce the use of animals for scientific procedures. These 3Rs (Replace, Reduce and Refine) runs like a thread through the Directive. Thus, EU's member states must ensure that live animals shall not be used when a scientifically satisfactory method or testing strategy not entailing the use of live animals is available (Chapter 1 Article 4, 13). Further development, validation and implementation of the 3Rs is promoted by the establishment of a Union reference laboratory for the validation of alternative methods (EURL ECVAM, 2015). The member states shall support the reference laboratory by promoting alternative methods at national level (Chapter V Article 47, 48).

The Directive sets minimum standards for animal protection (housing and care as well as the use of the animals) for the member states to implement in the national legislations. The member states had to implement the Directive into the national legislations by the end of 2012. After the date of publication of the Directive, the member states are not allowed to enforce stricter national legislation than that of the Directive. They could, however, ensure a continuous more extensive level of animal protection by keeping stricter national provisions. This could only be done if the stricter legislation was already in force before the Directive was published (Chapter I Article 2). To ensure that the member states comply with the set minimum standards of animal protection, regular risk-based inspections are required (Chapter IV Article 34).

Similar to the earlier Directive, all vertebrate animals including cyclostomes used for the purposes of basic research, higher education and training are covered by the present Directive. Based on evidence of sentience in cephalopods, these invertebrates are now also covered, and the scope was further widened to also include mammalian foetuses in their last third of development, since they are at risk of experiencing pain and suffering (Chapter I Article 1).

The Directive applies to animals that are used for scientific or educational purposes that are subjected to pain, suffering, distress or lasting harm equivalent to or higher than that caused by the insertion of a needle in accordance with good veterinary practice (Chapter I Article 3).

5.2.2.1 *Breeding Specifically for the Use in Procedures*
The use of certain animal species is specifically regulated in the Directive. The commonly used rodents and zebrafish, rabbits, cats and dogs as well as the non-human primates and some species of frogs have to be specifically bred for use in procedures (Chapter II Article 10). Research on great apes and other non-human primates should only be allowed for the purposes of preserving the species or when studying life-threatening, debilitating conditions that endanger human beings. The use of primates should only be chosen if there are no other alternatives to achieve the aims of the procedures (Chapter II Article 8).

Stray and feral animals should not be used in procedures, and animals taken from the wild shall not be used for scientific studies unless an exemption has been granted. The exemption shall only be given if the purpose of the procedure cannot be achieved by the use of an animal which has been bred for use in procedures. When animals are captured in the wild, the capturing procedure must be carried out by competent persons and it must be done with care, so that the animals are not caused any avoidable pain, suffering, distress or lasting harm (Chapter II Article 9,11).

5.2.2.2 *License to Perform Research, Requirements for Personnel and Educational Demands*
In order to get a license to do research with animals, European scientists must be adequately educated and trained (Chapter IV Article 23). This is done by participating in specific training covering theory and practice aiming to provide knowledge and skills to integrate the 3Rs into their research. To maintain or renew this license, subsequent

continuous professional development is required. Within the scientific community there is an increasing discussion of animal-related methodologies in preclinical research, much of which is focussed on ensuring clinically relevant and reliable results, but also including questions of good practice and the 3Rs in research. This has led to the publication of various sets of guidelines by researchers for researchers, as is further discussed in Section 5.5.

Further, there must always be at least one member of staff who is responsible for overseeing the welfare and care of the animals in the establishment as well as ensuring the education of the staff. Staff involved in caring for the animals, handling, planning, capturing or performing research must be adequately educated and trained until they have demonstrated the requisite competence. They must be educated and proven competent to perform their tasks before the research starts. Furthermore, the staff must be continuously trained (Chapter IV Article 24). For further guidance, see European Commission (2014a).

5.2.2.3 *Project Evaluation and Authorization*
All users of animals for scientific purposes must be authorized and registered by a so-called competent authority (Chapter IV Article 20), e.g. the authority(ies) in a member state responsible for regulating animal research. Projects must pass an ethical evaluation to receive authorization to use animals in research or teaching. The use of the animals will then have to be evaluated and justified in relation to the societal, scientific or educational purpose of the project. The project should be designed so as to enable procedures to be carried out in compliance with the requirement of the 3Rs (Russell and Burch, 1959). The evaluation of the project shall be performed in an impartial manner and the evaluation process must be transparent. The evaluation shall weigh the predicted societal and scientific benefits or educational value of the project against the suffering and harm the study infer to the animals. Furthermore, the evaluation shall verify that the project is designed to enable procedures being carried out in the most

humane and environmentally sensitive manner possible (Chapter IV Article 38). All projects are assessed regarding the degree of severity of the procedures involved and classified as 'non-recovery', 'mild', moderate' or 'severe'. No projects should be allowed that involve severe pain, suffering or distress that is likely to be long-lasting and cannot be ameliorated (Chapter III Article 15). The ethical evaluation shall also determine whether the project should be evaluated retrospectively, concerning the animal welfare and outcome of the study. For all projects, a non-technical project summary shall be published by the competent authority, to facilitate for the general public to have insight into the research performed (Chapter IV Article 39, 43).

5.2.2.4 *Animal Welfare Bodies*

All establishments that use animals for research must set up an Animal Welfare Body which shall include the person who is responsible for animal welfare and care and, in the case of a user, a scientific member. The animal welfare body shall also receive input from the designated veterinarian. The primary task of this body is giving advice on animal welfare issues, as well as the outcome of animal welfare in projects. The body should also foster a climate of care and provide tools for the practical application and timely implementation of recent technical and scientific developments in relation to the principles of replacement, reduction and refinement, in order to enhance the lifetime experience of the animals. The advice given by the animal welfare body should be properly documented and open to scrutiny during inspections by the competent authority (Chapter IV Article 26, 27). For further guidance, see European Commission (2014b).

5.2.2.5 *Reuse and Setting Free*

Member states shall ensure that an animal may only be reused in a new procedure provided that the actual severity of the previous procedures was 'mild' or 'moderate' and that the animal's general state of health and well-being has been fully restored. Veterinary advice shall be taken into account regarding the lifetime experience of the animal (Chapter II Article 16).

Member states may allow animals used in procedures to be returned to a suitable habitat appropriate to the species, provided that the state of health of the animal allows it and that there is no danger to public health, animal health or the environment (Chapter II Article 19).

In the following part of this chapter we describe the ethical review system, called project evaluation in the Directive 2010/63/EU, in some detail, as well as the development of this interdisciplinary review.

5.2.3 Review of Animal Experiments in Europe

It is nearly forty years since the first committees were established in Europe to review the ethical acceptability of research using animals. An important driver for the establishment of these committees was the recognition that animal research poses ethical challenges and that scientists need to be responsible and accountable for their actions. Research ethics committees for studies involving human subjects have been integral to good practice for the conduct of human research since the 1960s. Sweden was the first European country to introduce the obligatory ethics review process for research with animals in 1979. Since then, most other European countries have implemented different systems for ethics review, many of which involve evaluation by a multidisciplinary committee.

A working group established by the Federation of European Laboratory Animal Science Associations (FELASA) reviewed the methods and experiences of the ethics review process in 20 European countries in the early 2000s. This group reported that in 16 of these countries, national legislation required prior ethical review of all regulated scientific uses of animals. The report showed considerable variation in how ethics review was done in different countries (Smith *et al.*, 2007). For example, there was variation between countries regarding whether or not ethical review was legally required and/or binding, who performs the ethical review and how ethical decisions were made.

In Directive 2010/63/EU, the process through which projects are assessed and decisions made is termed 'project evaluation' and not 'ethics review', and there is also no reference to ethics committees. However, in line with language convention and practice in most EU member states, we will in this chapter use the terms 'ethics review' and 'animal ethics committees'. Whereas Directive 2010/63/EU is more specific than previous legislation was, the requirements for project evaluation are still very general, leaving it largely up to individual member states to define the structure within which the ethics review takes place, the content of the review and the composition of the committees. As a consequence, there is great variation in how reviews are organized and by whom projects are reviewed (Olsson *et al.*, 2016). In this chapter we provide an overview and reflections based on existing information in regulatory documents and scholarly literature.

5.2.3.1 *Structure Within Which the Ethics Review Takes Place*
According to Article 36, projects must be evaluated and authorized in advance by competent authorities. Each member state is to designate one or more competent authorities, or may designate bodies other than the public authorities if they have the expertise and infrastructure and no conflict of interests (Figure 5.1). In some countries, the entity performing the ethics review also has the power to authorize projects, whereas in others the ethics review produces a recommendation for the entity emitting the authorization. Ethics review may be carried out by the competent authorities (e.g. Belgium) or by other bodies (e.g. United Kingdom, Hungary), at local (e.g. Germany), regional (e.g. Sweden) or national (e.g. Denmark) level. Previously, several countries used a system with ethics review by individual experts; however, this seems to be giving way to a wider use of committees. One-person review is generally advised against, since it strongly limits the possibility to bring in different perspectives and completely misses out on the strength of dialogue as a deliberation tool (EWG, 2013).

Summary of the legal requirements of the Directive

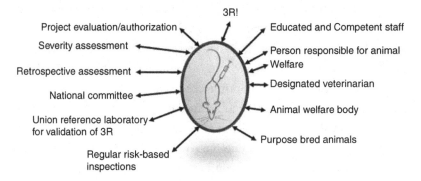

FIGURE 5.1 Overview sketch of the legal requirements surrounding the research animals in the EU.

Source: Original picture by Katarina Cvek.

5.2.3.2 *Content of Ethics Review*

In Directive 2010/63/EU, Article 38 specifies which aspects are to be assessed in the project evaluation and requires it to include an evaluation of the benefit, an assessment of 3Rs compliance, an assessment of the severity and a harm-benefit analysis. In most countries, these aspects were part of the ethics review process already before the revised legislation.

However, the FELASA working group reported that in some countries the review process focussed only on harms to animals and how to minimize them (Smith *et al.*, 2007). In practice, the focus on refinement to reduce harm may be even stronger. In their review of the minutes of Swedish animal ethics committee meetings, Hau and colleagues found that committees approved most applications as submitted, and when modifications were required, these were mainly for refinement of methods (Hagelin *et al.*, 2003; Hau *et al.*, 2001).

According to the FELASA report in 2005, five countries did not include a harm-benefit analysis in the ethics review before this became a legal requirement (Smith *et al.*, 2007). The harm-benefit analysis is probably the most challenging and arguably also the most controversial aspect of ethics review. Several recent initiatives have been set up to tackle this challenge. One of this is the American Association for Laboratory Animal Science - Federation of European Laboratory Animal Science Associations (AALAS-FELASA) Working Group on Harm-Benefit Analysis of Animal Studies (Laber *et al.*, 2016), which recognized the harm-benefit analysis as 'the cornerstone of ethical evaluation, as it will determine if the use of animals is justified'. Based on a review of different formalized approaches to harm-benefit weighing, including existing mathematical, graphic and algorithm models Laber et al. developed a process-oriented model for harm-benefit analysis within project authorization. In a similar vein, in Austria, the Federal Ministry for Science and Research asked scientists to set up criteria for the evaluation of animal experiments 'in order to enable an objective harm-benefit analysis' (Messerli – Research Institute, 2012).

However, whether the harm-benefit analysis is really an appropriate component of the ethics review has also been questioned. One option would be that the ethics review focuses on harm reduction only, or alternatively to restrict full harm-benefit analyses to experiments causing (or judged likely to cause) severe harm to the animals (Vieira de Castro and Olsson, 2015). Although benefits have a core role in discussions in AEC (see Chapter 1), there is undoubtedly an inherent difficulty in assessing benefits. Whereas harms will generally predictably happen and within the course of the project, benefits are uncertain and much more distant in time. Recommendations for benefit assessment therefore often focus on standard measures of scientific potential and quality, such as how original, timely and realistic the objectives are, if there is replication of previous work and how the proposed work relates to other work in the field as well as experimental design, researcher competence, the appropriateness and quality of facilities and how the results will be communicated (Smith *et al.*, 2007). Nevertheless, several current proposals argue that wider societal benefit should also be considered (European Commission, 2015). One recently suggested method that seeks to avoid the harm-benefit dualism is to ascribe ethical weights to different clinical signs or research procedures in order to estimate acceptable ethical cost. One key question in ethical review supposedly facilitated by such an approach is how to balance refinement versus reduction (Ringblom *et al.*, 2017).

5.2.3.3 *Expertise and Representation*

Whereas the Directive does not specify who should participate in the ethics review, Article 38 defines the expertise that must be considered:

(a) the areas of scientific use for which animals will be used including replacement, reduction and refinement in the respective areas;

(b) experimental design, including statistics where appropriate;

(c) veterinary practice in laboratory animal science or wildlife veterinary practice where appropriate;

(d) animal husbandry and care, in relation to the species that are intended to be used.

A multidisciplinary committee is perhaps the most common approach to ensure that this range of expertise is involved in the review. Participation in ethical review processes varied between the 17 FELASA member countries in 2005 (Smith *et al.*, 2007). Considerable variation between member states as regards committee composition remains under Directive 2010/63/EU both in terms of the types of expertise and representation involved and the balance between different expertise or representation. The most consistent participants in ethics review are scientists and veterinarians. Other technical expertise includes – in some countries – specialists on design and analysis of experiments and on alternatives to animal experiments as well as legal and ethics experts. In some countries, the committee is fully composed of technical experts, whereas other countries include one or more members from outside the research community, most commonly representatives of animal protection NGOs. Only one country (Sweden) has a committee with as many lay representatives as technical experts.

The rationale for involving lay persons may be to ensure that perspectives from outside the research environment is brought into the decision-making over animal research as well as to increase transparency, thereby raising the legitimacy of decisions. However studies show that lay persons play a very limited role in the ethics committee discussion. Researchers examining how the effectiveness of Canadian animal ethics committees was influenced by committee composition and dynamics, found a bias towards institutional or scientific interests (Schuppli and Fraser, 2007). Even in Sweden where experts are not in majority in the animal ethics committees, their technocratic voice dominates discussion and decision-making (Ideland, 2009, Röcklinsberg 2015).

5.2.3.4 *Wider Implications of the Ethics Review*

Ethics review as part of animal experimentation legislation should respond to societal concerns over the use of animals in experiments. In this context, ethics review will also interact with other aspects of legislation in ways which have implications for both science and society.

Although harm-benefit analysis has always been exercised as a tool for moral justification in animal research regulation, questions on its role in the authorization process have appeared more recently when ongoing research has been blocked by ethics committee decisions, such as in the following example from Germany.

Andreas Kreiter at the University of Bremen used macaques to study cognitive processes in the mammalian brain in 2007 when his project expired and he was told it was not to be renewed. Referring to 'changed societal values', the authority argued that the experiments were 'ethically unjustified' because they addressed long-term scientific questions rather than helped to develop specific medical therapies (Schiermeier, 2008). Although the terms of benefits or relevance of research were not explicitly referred to, these were likely the underlying reason behind the refusal to renew the project license. After a long legal procedure, in 2014 the Federal Administrative Court (which has upheld the previous court decision) ruled that authorities had no entitlement to assess the ethical justification of an experiment, but were obliged to approve an application if all formalities were complied with (Ruhdel *et al.*, 2014).

This case illustrates several issues of relevance for the ethics review. First, it shows that if not well embedded in the authorization process, ethics review may be legally overturned. Second, it illustrates the problem of an obscure harm-benefit analysis, with conflicting expectations between different stakeholders. The ethics committee considered it their mission to evaluate benefit and to halt the experiment on basis of this part of the assessment, but this was clearly not the expectation of the applying scientist or of his peers who supported him and expressed consternation over the decision. However, this case is far from representative: the vast majority of research objectives are in practice considered sufficient to justify animal use and grant approval of applications.

Article 38 (4) of the Directive requires that the project evaluation process be transparent. Transparency of public institutions means that citizens should be able to find out what is going on inside public offices and it is generally supposed to make institutions and their office-holders trusted and trustworthy. Within the present European legislation, the two main methods of safeguarding and encouraging openness in animal research are the recognition of right to information and the legally binding publication of non-technical summaries.

The recognition of the right to access public information (freedom of information laws, or FOI) has become a cornerstone of transparency in democratic countries. These laws establish a 'right-to-know' about any legal process by which requests may be made for government-held information, which shall be received freely or at minimal cost, barring standard exceptions. FOI legislation can be used to assess the practices of governments with regard to both their conduct and their regulation of animal experiments, including application of the 3Rs. However, only individual requests are allowed, and the scope of questions is limited, preventing this method from being used for an overall evaluation of research animal protection. Considering the need to protect personal security and intellectual property access to detailed information about animal research is controversial.

Directive 2010/63/EU includes a requirement for applications to include a non-technical summary outlining the process and objective of the research project (including why animals are being used, what species is being used and why it has been chosen, the number of animals required and the benefit of using animals for the research proposed) in a simple manner. If the application is approved, an anonymous version of this lay summary will be published on the Internet, similar to what is already practised in Denmark and the United Kingdom. However, a study of non-technical summaries found that these tend to overemphasize benefits and overlook animal suffering, and therefore questioned whether the publication of non-technical summaries will provide a sufficient level of transparency to eliminate public concerns (Phillips and Jennings, 2008).

5.3 REGULATION AND ETHICS REVIEW IN NORTH AMERICA

In North America, Animal Ethics Committees (AECs) play a vital role in the governance of animal research. This section outlines how AECs are situated in the broader governance of animal-based research in Canada and the United States. Ethical challenges and shortcomings of current AECs are discussed and recommendations on how to improve the functioning of AECs in North America are put forward. The fact that some themes overlap with issues dealt with elsewhere in the book shows not only the importance of discussing challenges in each research context, but also the universal character of these challenges.

5.3.1 *Governance in Canada*

There is no national legislation regulating the use of animals in science in Canada, and private companies that are self-funded are not required to comply with national guidelines (though they may apply to be certified and inspected). However, the use of animals (defined as non-human vertebrates and cephalopods) in publicly funded science is overseen by a national organization called the Canadian Council on Animal Care (CCAC). The CCAC aims to act in the

Table 5.1 *Canadian Council on Animal Care approach to advancing animal ethics and care in science.*

1	Guidelines and policies based on science-informed standards
2	National mandated educational curriculum
3	Regular assessment and certification of institutional animal use programs – Certificate of Good Animal Practice
4	Collection and publication of statistics on national animal use
5	Ethical review of animal projects by local institutional Animal Ethics Committees

Source: Original table by Catherine Schuppli and Elisabeth Ormandy.

interests of Canadians to 'advance animal ethics and care in science' (CCAC, 2015). The CCAC achieves these goals in a number of ways (Table 5.1). It sets science-informed standards through the creation of guidelines and policies for animal care and use in science. The CCAC has also created a national curriculum of education mandated for all animal users. In addition to provision of resources such as guidelines and educational materials, the CCAC carries out regular assessment and certification of the institutional animal use programs at individual institutions under its purview. At the local level, institutions are required to provide information on their use of animals: numbers and species of animals, purpose of use and the numbers of animals exposed to four levels of pain and distress called the 'Categories of Invasiveness'. These categories go from least invasive (Category B) to most invasive (Category E) and outline the potential harm that might come to animals during a scientific procedure (CCAC 1991). The CCAC collates this information and publishes annual reports, made available to the public. In addition, each institution under the CCAC program is required to have an Animal Ethics Committee (known as the Animal Care Committee, ACC) that oversees animal use within their institution, ensuring that animal-based research complies with the CCAC national standards.

Although there is no national legislation, CCAC compliance is achieved in a variety of ways. Currently, 8 of the 13 Canadian provinces and territories make compliance with national CCAC standards a requirement under provincial law. In all regions, receipt of federal research funds by any institution is contingent upon compliance with CCAC standards. The CCAC has developed publically recognized trademarks, certificate of 'Good Animal Practice' (GAP ®), which are awarded to any institution, public or private, which meet CCAC standards as determined by assessments. For Canadian researchers receiving certain US funding, CCAC standards are recognized by the American Association for the Assessment and Accreditation of Laboratory of Animal Care International (AAALAC International, see below) as equivalent to US standards.

5.3.2 *Governance in the United States*

Oversight of laboratory animal care and use in the United States is multi-faceted, provided by two government bodies and one private, non-profit association. All require the appointment of an AEC (called Institutional Animal Care and Use Committee (IACUC). IACUCs in the United States are intended to serve similar functions to the ACCs in Canada.

The United States Department of Agriculture (USDA) implements and enforces the national Animal Welfare Act (AWA, from 1976) through the development of the Animal Welfare Regulations (CFR (Code of Federal Regulations), 1985). The Act covers 'warm-blooded' animals used in research, teaching or testing but excludes 'birds, rats of the genus *Rattus*, and mice of the genus *Mus*' and 'livestock or poultry used or intended for use as food or fiber, or livestock or poultry used or intended for use for improving animal nutrition, breeding, management, or production efficiency, or for improving the quality of food or fiber'.

The Office of Laboratory Animal Welfare (OLAW) is located within the National Institutes of Animal Health (NIH) and is responsible for guidance on and for monitoring compliance with Public Health Service (PHS) Policy on Humane Care and Use of Laboratory Animals (OLAW, 2002). This policy requires an animal care and use program with an Animal Ethics Committee. All PHS-supported research, such as NIH, Centre for Disease Control and Food and Drug Administration funded projects, falls under OLAW jurisdiction. PHS covers 'live, vertebrate animal[s] used or intended for use in research, research training, experimentation, or biological testing or for related purposes' (OLAW, 2002). Therefore, PHS covers species not legally covered by the Animal Welfare Act. OLAW uses CCAC guidelines as reference materials. In the case of research funded by NIH to Canadian researchers, OLAW requires a 'Foreign Animal Welfare Assurance' which includes questions related to compliance with relevant CCAC standards.

The Association for Assessment and Accreditation of Laboratory Animal Care International (AAALAC) is a voluntary accreditation system that any institution can choose to participate in, in addition to their required national compliance (Hamm *et al.*, 1995). AAALAC bases its standards on Guide for the Care and Use of Laboratory Animals (NRC, 2011), the Guide for the Care and Use of Agricultural Animals in Research and Teaching (FASS, 2010) and The European Convention for the Protection of Vertebrate Animals used for Experimental and other Scientific Purposes (Council of Europe, 1986). AAALAC covers 'traditional laboratory animals, farm animals, wildlife, and aquatic animals. Nontraditional animals, inclusive of invertebrate species, are also included where they are relevant to the unit's mission' (AAALAC, 2015).

In the United States, the USDA collects and publishes national statistics on numbers of animals for species covered by the Animal Welfare Act. Estimates are provided for rodents, birds, fish, reptiles or amphibians. Within institutions, the Animal Ethics Committee accounts for numbers of animals in their research review process, but this is not typically published.

5.3.3 *Animal Ethics Committees: Tasks and Structure in North America*

Canadian and US AECs are similar in their composition, processes and responsibilities. The AECs in North America are located within an institution, and the relevant governing bodies require that membership include a selection of members drawn from within the institution: scientists and/or teachers experienced in animal care and use, veterinarians, non-animal-users, non-scientists, students and animal technical staff, together with people independent of the institution who can represent local community interests (CFR, 1985; OLAW, 2002; CCAC, 2006).

A major function of the Animal Ethics Committee is to review all proposed research involving animals at the institution, judge it on the basis of its ethical acceptability and minimize harms to animals in various ways. Review of protocols and committee process is carried out according to guidance documents published by the relevant governing body. In all cases, AEC decisions are guided by the 3Rs (Russell and Burch, 1959). Canadian policy and the AWA, AAALAC in the United States mandate that approval of animal-based research be determined by balancing the potential benefits of the research against the harms to animals (CCAC, 1997; CFR, 1985; NRC, 2011). This includes minimizing pain from experimental procedures as well as considering reduced well-being resulting from inappropriate housing, care and handling.

To ensure acceptable care and use by animal users within their institution, AECs are also involved in a number of activities related to oversight of the entire animal use program. They organize and operate educational opportunities. These range from basic courses in rodent biology and husbandry to specialized training based on the needs of researchers. In addition, AEC members are involved in regular inspection of animal facilities in their institution. For example, OLAW requires IACUC inspection of all animal facilities every six months (OLAW, 2002).

5.3.4 *Key Challenges to the Effectiveness of North American Animal Ethics Committees*

5.3.4.1 *Committee Composition*
Schuppli and Fraser (2007) found that AEC effectiveness is influenced by committee composition and dynamics, recruitment of members,

workload, participation level and member turnover. They found a potential bias towards institutional or research interests versus interests of research subjects and the community resulting from (1) a preponderance of institutional members, especially scientists; (2) committee dynamics and poor leadership by chairpersons that prevented full participation of community and minority members; (3) community members being affiliated with the institution; and (4) some members' motivation for joining the AEC to pursue agendas other than the committee mandate. In addition, thoroughness of review could be affected by excessive workload or inadequate review and low turnover of members, limiting new ideas and risking indoctrination. Based on the problems identified, this research identified potential solutions as well as provided a basis for developing standards for performance assessment, which is important for assuring quality and performance of a system for protection of research subjects. It is suggested that attention to committee composition might improve AEC deliberations and that lessons can be learned from other countries with different committee compositions. Overall, evidence-based governance will be essential for addressing some of these challenges.

5.3.4.2 *Animal Ethics Committee Procedures*

Ethical Justification of Research Ethically justifying animal-based research requires, among other things, that there is promise of benefits, that the research is scientifically valid, that harms to research subjects are minimized, and that the benefits outweigh harms. Ensuring that these ethical criteria are met is achieved at a variety of levels ranging from individual researchers, to peer review by committees in granting agencies, to AECs, to public officials, scientists, patient advocates and others who make decisions about research priorities, budgets and policies. The roles and relationships between these different groups are complex, with some groups focusing on particular ethical criteria more than others. In some cases it is unclear who is covering which criteria and who should be responsible for covering which criteria. For example, empirical research on AECs has shown that when they review proposed research that has been funded by a granting agency, members often take expert peer review by granting agencies as an assurance of both technical merit and social value without further need for weighing benefits against harms, and consequently the AEC members limit their review process to minimizing harms to animals (APC, 2003; Schuppli, 2011). They do this because they trust scientific peer review committees of granting agencies to ensure that the proposed research produces social benefit and is scientifically valid. Thus, the question of whether the benefits are sufficient to outweigh the harms is not necessarily addressed.

The promise of benefits and a favourable harm-benefit ratio are essential elements of arguments for justifying the involvement of animals in research. For research to be considered ethical, it is not sufficient to simply ensure that animals are used and treated humanely. Yet, it is unclear how much AECs go beyond identifying and minimizing harm. In the United States, Brody (1998) suggests, committees only focus on minimizing harm. There is a need to sort out some basic issues about how to assess the ethical justification of research. To what extent do (or can) AECs assess social benefits, scientific validity and harm-benefit ratios? Should they do so? Could changes in policy help them do it better? What are the relative roles of granting agency and ethics committees in covering the different elements of harm-benefit assessments? Could expert peer review committees change their practices to meet the needs of ethics committees, leaving ethics committees to focus only on harm assessment? Could (or should) research using animals be justified at the specific or the aggregate level? Which of these options will likely meet public expectations of providing adequate protection for animals and humans involved in research?

One possible solution would be to provide AECs with more guidance on their role in meeting the expectations of policy. In part, this may require clarifying policy so that it provides a fuller description of what elements should be considered in decisions about the ethical justification of research. By explicitly breaking down decisions about justification into different components, committee members may be better equipped to assess whether the research is ethically justified, and perhaps be able to identify whether or not peer review by granting agencies has already covered any of these components.

Policy may also need to clarify the role that expert peer review by granting agencies plays in these decisions. Grant reviewers often assess the expected benefits of proposals but generally do not evaluate harm to animals or consider the 3Rs. Thus, it seems that peer reviews at the granting agency level may sometimes miss key components of AEC's evaluations, thus making it even more important for AECs to consider these issues. However, AEC members may rely on expert peer review because they feel ill-equipped to make cost-benefit assessments. Thus, we need to ask what AECs can reasonably be expected to evaluate.

I. Technical Merit: First, it seems reasonable to expect scientist members on an AEC to be able to assess technical merit of proposals at least at the level of appropriate experimental design, statistics and appropriateness of the animal model.

II. Harms and the 3Rs: With appropriate training, committee members should be able to apply the 3Rs. Similarly, members should be able to evaluate harms to animals, although some members (the veterinarian, animal technicians and possibly community members from the humane movement) will be more skilled at this. However, there are difficulties with assessing harms; Schuppli and Fraser (2005) found that members varied in their interpretation of pain and what they considered harmful, as well as beliefs about the moral significance of pain and suffering, with different interpretations resulting in different views about the need for and degree of pain mitigation.

Notions such as pain, suffering and distress are greatly debated by scientists and philosophers, and there may be conceptual confusion at the national or policy level. As a result, the ethical significance of these concepts is open to question, making the challenge that AEC members face very great. Lack of clarity in the meaning of these concepts makes it hard to apply them to harm-benefit assessments in a standard manner.

III. Social Value: Social value may be the most difficult for AEC members to assess. Some scientists may be able to assess social value for proposals that are in their own field of expertise, but community members would certainly have difficulty doing so.

Predicting potential benefits of research is notoriously difficult, yet it is the cornerstone of arguments for the justification of the use of animals in research. In some cases, the benefits used to justify experiments seem quite clear. For example, safety testing of products provides clear benefit to the public by helping to eliminate unsafe products from the marketplace. On the other hand, predicting health applications of fundamental research and the probability of achieving those desired benefits is inevitably more speculative (Dresser, 2001; Jennings and Silcock, 1995). Therefore, such research is not easily accommodated within a cost-benefit assessment. Since benefits are a key element of assessing justification, how can we make this process more effective?

If AECs are not able to predict benefits, then one solution would be to provide information where possible. Perhaps investigators could be asked to describe the benefits expected to flow from the work. Investigators could be asked to rate the importance of the contribution (as is done in the Animals Scientific Procedures, Act 1986 [Home Office, 1986] in the United Kingdom). If the research contributes to fundamental knowledge, then how important is the contribution to that field? If the research contributes to some clinical application, then how significant is the health problem? What is the likelihood that this research will contribute to this clinical application and how long might it take to realize the benefit? Breaking the assessments of benefits down into constituent components should serve to make explicit the kinds of issues AECs should consider, and highlight points of uncertainty or disagreement in discussions.

However, benefits may be overestimated by investigators. In a research culture that is highly competitive for funding it is likely that investigators will emphasize and amplify the value and expected benefits of their work. This makes it particularly critical for independent assessments of the benefits of the proposed research.

Scientific peer reviewers at the granting agency may be better equipped than AECs are to provide an objective evaluation of potential benefits. Therefore, an alternative solution would be to have scientific peer reviewers provide the necessary information, as outlined above, so that AECs could carry out their cost-benefit assessments.

If scientific peer reviewers at granting agencies were able to assess expected benefits, then another approach would be to rely on such reviews to also assess the ethical justification of the work. In this case, peer review by granting committees would have to change their practice to include a harm-benefit evaluation. This might require changing the composition of peer review committees to include members with expertise in evaluating animal harm, as well community members. In this case, AECs could accept that a positive peer review establishes that benefits outweigh harms and focus only on harm.

Finally, given the problems with cost-benefit assessments, perhaps the case for justification of animal research can be made at an aggregate level. That is, we could ask whether the overall benefits accruing from animal research in general are sufficient to justify the current level of use of animals. In this scenario the decision-making system dealing with research priorities, budgets and policies would serve to identify worthy areas of research in a process involving public officials, scientists, patient advocates and others (Dresser, 2001). The AEC is then exempted from having to consider the (often imponderable) likely future benefits of a given experiment, and instead their only role would be to minimize harms to animals. Even with shortcomings in AEC and scientific peer review, and with challenges involved in setting research priorities, perhaps the combination of these checks and balances in the governance system will ensure public confidence in the mechanisms and processes to ensure justified animal use.

Decision-Making Approaches In a study of US AECs, Plous and Herzog (2001) found inconsistency in decision-making across AECs. Differences are also present within a committee (Schuppli, 2011). For example, community members tend to use emotion and moral intuition in their approach to decision-making, more than other members. Scientists tended to be more willing than other members to trust the expert peer review process to assess technical merit and social benefits, and also to trust investigators to implement Reduction and Replacement. Third, animal technicians tended to show the lowest level of trust that investigators would carry out procedures as they had written them in their application form. In addition to the type of harm-benefit assessment prescribed in policies, other styles of decision-making may strengthen the AEC review process by accepting a greater diversity of views.

Bureaucratic Compliance The administration of researchers needed to comply with institutional oversight requirements has been described as 'bureaucratic', 'burdensome' and 'excessive' (NSB, 2014; Ormandy, 2012; Ormandy et al., 2013). It is argued that the administrative workload of scientists is increasing but the requirements are ineffective and a 'waste of taxpayer's money' (NSB, 2014). In this case, it is important to continually evaluate the effectiveness of AECs and to develop performance-based standards.

5.4 REGULATION AND REVIEW OF ANIMAL EXPERIMENTS IN ASIA, LATIN AMERICA AND OCEANIA

In both Asia and Latin America there are countries with regulated systems (e.g. India and South Korea in Asia; Brazil, Mexico and Uruguay in Latin America) while others have no regulatory framework yet. As in other geographical areas described in this chapter, when regulated systems exist, they may be based on ethical review bodies at public authority level, at institutional level, or combination of both. However, it is not uncommon that some of the systems are not fully implemented at ground level. On the other side, the generally increasing awareness is leading to the establishment of voluntary ethical review processes in other countries lacking regulations or guidelines. Systems in place in Oceania are well developed and implemented.

5.4.1 Asia

A number of Asian countries have already developed specific regulations, including India, South Korea, Taiwan, Malaysia, Philippines and Singapore (Guillén, 2014). The Chinese system depends more on provincial laws and the Japanese on the Guidelines by the Science Council.

India has a regulated system based on the Prevention of Cruelty to Animals Act from 1960 (Ministry of Environment and Forest I 1960) and more recent updates (Ministry of Environment and Forest I 1998a; b; 2001) that combine central and institutional activities. There is a central Committee for the Purpose of Control and Supervision of Experiments on Animals (CPCSEA) having general oversight functions, while main ethical review functions on the ground are assigned to and implemented by Institutional Animal Ethics Committees (IAEC). Each IAEC has eight members, five of them from the Institution (a biological scientist, the scientist in charge of the animal facility, the named veterinarian and two scientists from a different biological discipline) and the other three (the main nominee, the scientist from outside the institution and a nonscientific socially aware member) are appointed by the CPCSEA. The CPCSEA has to approve some of the decisions taken by the IAECs.

The Chinese system is more recent and comes from the statute promulgated in 1982 that was expanded and updated in 2006 (MOST,

2006). Government regulations are implemented through provincial laws. Institutions must establish a Welfare and Ethics Committee with the following composition: staff from management, scientific and technical personnel, professional veterinary staff and external lay members. The functioning of these committees may vary depending on the provincial laws. A proposed draft on a new government law on animal protection contains a chapter that focuses on laboratory animals and proposes the constitution of a national ethics committee and also of provincial ethics committee to supervise and harmonize principles and guidelines.

In Japan the Institutional Animal Care and Use Committees (IACUC) are not legally mandatory, but are proposed by the Guidelines for Proper Conduct of Animal Experiments (Japan Science Council, 2006) that serve as a reference or model for institutions when developing their own self-regulated systems. According to these guidelines, the IACUC members are nominated by the president of each research institution and include researchers conducting animal experiments, laboratory animal specialists and other persons of knowledge and experience. In these guidelines there is no request for the attending veterinarian to be a member of the IACUC. The proposed activities of the IACUC are limited to protocol review, and other activities (i.e. post-approval monitoring or review of the animal care and use program) depend on each institutional commitment.

The Animal Welfare Act in South Korea requires institutions to establish an IACUC with defined functions including follow-up on projects (Ministry of Agriculture FaRA, 1991). Membership is between 3 and 15 members, including a specialized veterinarian and an external animal welfare specialist.

Ethical review is based on IACUCs in other Asian countries with specific legislation such as Taiwan, Malaysia, Philippines and Singapore. A number of institutions in countries with no specific legislation have established IACUCs on a voluntary basis.

All these examples show that when legislation is in place in Asian countries, ethical review is performed mainly by IACUCs.

Governments usually lack the expertise and resources to perform an efficient control, so they pragmatically have to rely on local bodies. Only in very few cases may central authorities play a role. As in other countries around the world, relying on local bodies to perform ethical review, a potential conflict of interest may happen when these bodies do not have external input and/or the government oversight is poor. On the other hand, IACUCs may be the only way to achieve a real ethical review, and they are frequently adopted on a voluntary basis in countries with no legislation in place. Therefore, the institutional commitment is paramount to ensure the ethical review is performed appropriately.

5.4.2 Latin America

In Latin America the countries with specific legislation on the care and use of laboratory animals are Brazil (Presidência da República CC, 2008), Mexico (Secretaría de Agricultura, 2001) and Uruguay (Government of Uruguay, 2009). In other countries there are some regulations in this field as part of more general animal protection laws.

In Brazil, Mexico and Uruguay the ethical review process is mandatory and operated locally, governed by IACUCs called Comissão de Ética no Uso de Animais (CEUA) in Brasil and Comité Institucional para el Cuidado y Uso de Animales de Laboratorio (CICUAL) in most of the other Latin American countries. Composition are very similar and include a veterinarian, researchers/teachers in relevant areas and an external member representative of animal protection society (in the case of the Brazilian CEUA).

In other countries with no specific requirement, such as Chile, Colombia, Peru or Argentina, the establishment of CICUALs on a voluntary basis is very common. For example, in Chile and Colombia there are active networks of CICUALs at several research institutions and universities.

As in Asia, ethical review in Latin America depends on IACUCs, very similar in composition to the US IACUCs, either established as a legal requirement or on a voluntary basis. The difference is that lack of government resources and expertise in this field is even more dramatic. The most common problem is that CICUALs are not given the necessary authority by the institution, and quite frequently their activity is restricted to the prospective review of protocols.

5.4.3 *Oceania*

Although in Australia the legal responsibility for the welfare and use of animals in research lies with the animal welfare regulatory authority of each state or territory, which means the specific regulations differ among them, the Australian Code for the Care and Use of Animals for Scientific Purposes (NHMRC, 2013) serves as the main framework to which the different pieces of legislation adhere in terms of principles and guidelines. Part 6 of the New Zealand Animal Welfare Act (Government of New Zealand, 1999) establishes the legal requirements for ethical review in New Zealand.

The Australian Code is based upon the local Animal Ethics Committees (AEC). Membership must include at least one person of the following categories: a veterinarian with experience relevant to the activities of the institution (Category A); a qualified person with substantial recent experience in the use of animals in scientific or teaching activities (Category B); a person with demonstrable commitment to, and established experience in, furthering the welfare of animals, who is not employed by or otherwise associated with the institution, and who is not involved in the care and use of animals for scientific purposes (Category C); and a person who is both independent of the institution and has never been involved in the use of animals in scientific or teaching activities, either in employment or beyond their undergraduate education (Category D). The Code also recommends the appointment of persons responsible for the routine care of animals within the institution and persons with specific expertise to provide advice as required. To ensure the independence of the decision process, it is stated that where an AEC has more than four members, Categories C and D should represent no less than one third of the members.

Australian AECs are entrusted not only with protocol review functions but also with oversight and monitoring of animal care and use, including post-approval monitoring, and have the authority to intervene, recommend changes and even suspend animal activities if appropriate.

New Zealand AECs perform similar functions and must consist of at least four members: the institutional code-of-ethics holder (or a senior member appointed by the chief executive); a veterinarian; an external person not involved with the institution and not involved with animal use; and a person from the regional competent authority.

Again, it is evident that local bodies are responsible for ethical research also in Oceania, in this case as part of well-defined systems. It has been described how local bodies are responsible in general in Asia, Latin America and Oceania (Guillén, 2014). The involvement of competent authorities in the process is minimal or non-existent in many countries of Asia and Latin America due to lack of knowledge and resources. Therefore, the expertise and competence of such bodies are, along with the institutional commitment to provide them with authority, transparency and independence, the key to ensuring the implementation of appropriate ethical review processes.

5.5 GUIDELINES FOR RESEARCHERS BY RESEARCHERS

In February 1975 about 140 professionals working within the emerging field of recombinant DNA met at a conference in Asilomar, United States. The result of the meeting was a moratorium on creating organisms based on recombinant DNA until security procedures has been established. This has later been hailed as one of the prime examples of researchers taking their responsibilities towards society seriously. Another concerns the group of nuclear physicists led by Nobel Laurate Niels Bohr who after developing the nuclear bomb during the Second World War tried to influence the political system to harness the technology only for peaceful purposes. Possibly the biologists at the Asilomar meeting in 1975 thought back on the physicists from 30 years before and had that situation in mind when they decided to discuss if they should set up rules for their research before the cat was let out of the bag.

Within the world of laboratory animals one of the earliest and best-known examples of self-regulation by scientists is the 3Rs (see Section 3.3) developed by the two British scientists, William Russell and Rex Burch, in 1959. Since then many codes of conducts have been proposed by and for people working with lab animals. Self-regulation is thus not a new phenomenon and can be seen as part and parcel of a growing recognition of the unavoidable connection between the methods and results of scientific inquiry and the societal consequences (Figure 5.2; Guidelines for the Use of Animals, 1997).

One of the advantages of self-regulation in science as seen from the perspective of the researchers is that it can create win-win situations. Both with regard to the Asilomar Moratorium and the 3Rs, it is worth noting that they seem to be motivated not only by a sense of responsibility but also by a desire to be able to do the best research possible. By agreeing to the moratorium in 1975 the scientists showed the public that they took concerns regarding safety issues seriously and thereby perhaps avoided having a much stricter regulation imposed on them. The 3Rs are designed to ensure the welfare of the lab animals while warranting the best possible scientific outcome of the research. As long as that goes hand in hand with better animal welfare or using fewer animals, it is a win-win situation. Thus self-regulation can be a way of avoiding stricter societal regulation by ensuring responsible use of animals.

An advantage of self-regulation as seen from the perspective of society is that the regulation is based on the expert knowledge of the research community and therefore the best available understanding of the possible consequences for research methodologies of the regulation. Another advantage is that the values that the self-imposed regulation seeks to protect typically will be shared by the research community and therefore be considered worthy of protection.

An obvious problem with self-regulation is that the balancing of research interests and societal interests when done by the research

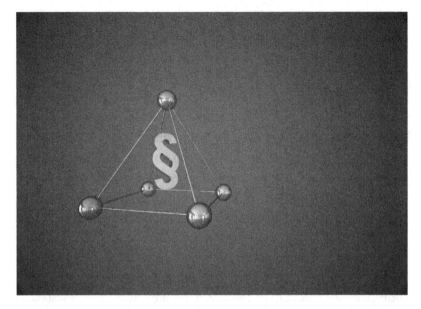

FIGURE 5.2 Self-regulation involves both individual ethical discernment and collective ethical reflection in order to ensure awareness of ethical responsibility for direct and indirect consequences of research.

Source: Image from Getty images

community easily becomes skewed towards placing as few limits on research as possible. Even though it is tempting to leave regulation in the hands of experts to get a neutral and objective result, this is not what happens. When decisions are left to experts, their values will be promoted. Another problem is that the control mechanisms of a self-regulatory system often are based primarily on trust and voluntary participation, and that the sanctions within self-regulatory systems rarely are as strict as those that imposed by society. It thus becomes both easier and less costly to transgress the rules.

As already mentioned, an early example of self-regulation within the area of animal research is the 3Rs that have been so successful as to have been implemented into the legislation of many countries and even international bodies such as the EU.

As examples of what self-regulation within this field can cover and how far-reaching it is in comparison with existing societal regulation, we have chosen to look first into two sets of guidelines for researcher self-regulation, both originating in Switzerland, and then to provide an overview of international guidelines.

5.5.1 General Ethical Guidelines for Research with Animals

Considering the high importance of biomedical research in Switzerland, 'Ethical Principles and Guidelines for Experiments on Animals (EPGE)' were written by the Swiss Academy of Medical Sciences and the Swiss Academy of Sciences in 1983 and declared binding as a code of conduct for all researchers and their scientific collaborators practising in Switzerland. These principles and guidelines are based on the perspective that experimentation on live animals is indispensable to resolve certain health problems on the one hand, while on the other hand the ethical principles of 'respect for life' and respect for the 'dignity of creation' demand that animals are protected. The Ethical Principles and Guidelines are based on the conviction that, as responsible persons, scientists should themselves define, implement and monitor the measures necessary to attain the best possible resolution of this conflict (Preamble).

A much more recent set of guidelines related to animal experiments developed by researchers is the international 'Basel Declaration' stating to be 'A call for more trust, transparency and communication on animal research' (The Basel Declaration, 2015). The Basel Declaration states that 'social and humanitarian challenges' posed by unsolved biomedical problems cannot be overcome without research using animals. It permits no demarcation line to be drawn between basic research and applied science, but declares that it 'is a continuum stretching from studies of fundamental physiological processes to an understanding of the principles of disease and the development of therapies'. Every attempt to get closer to fair solutions in handling (experimental) animals must be taken seriously and be weighed for its potential value. In the following, we will briefly compare these two sets of guidelines. Both emerge from researchers in Switzerland, but ethically relevant differences can be seen.

1. The Basel Declaration follows the Swiss Animal Protection Law, which is comparable with the Directive 2010/63/EU when it comes to animals in research. Different from EPGE, some of the Basel commitments focus on scientists' possibility to influence the public understanding of science, and to advise political decision makers and government authorities on 'issues of research involving animals and their welfare'. Hence these guidelines cover both animal welfare and researcher's possibility to communicate their own perspective to a broader public. This mirrors the background of each initiative. Whereas the Basel Declaration is a response to a discussion on improving scientists' openness about their work in order to gain public trust, the EPGE have a more philosophical approach taking the ethical dilemma of experimental medical research into account and highlight scientists' responsibility to define, implement and monitor the measures necessary to attain the best possible resolution of the ethical dilemma of animal research.

2. The point 5.2 of the EPGE is more far-reaching than most guidelines: 'Researchers employed in Switzerland shall refrain from carrying out experiments on animals abroad that contravene the Swiss animal welfare legislation and cannot be justified on the basis of these Ethical Principles and Guidelines and from participating in their implementation abroad.'

3. In general the Basel Declaration remains at law level, but exceeds it in one point: It encourages a free and transparent exchange to avoid unnecessary duplication of experiments. The EPGE is, however, again somewhat more demanding in this respect, stating (5.3): 'Persons involved in research … are also obliged to promote the exchange of information about the results of experiments on animals so as to avoid unnecessary experiments and, where applicable, to support the updating of regulations and methods.' This is also a stronger claim than laid down in the Directive 2010/63/EU, stating that unnecessary repetition should not be accepted in the ethical assessment/project evaluation process.

4. The Basel Declaration strongly invites representatives of animal welfare organizations to openly discuss all important questions with the scientists. In comparison, the EPGE regards it a duty of scientists to educate themselves on animal protection issues (5.4): 'Persons involved in scientific research are obliged to do further training in animal welfare

and to support the development of alternative research methods.'
Again we have that clear difference: the Declaration invites discussion,
whereas the EPGE demands from scientists to strongly consider the
implementation of alternatives.

As shown, the Basel Declaration poses less restrictions on the sign-
ees compared to what Swiss scientists imposed on themselves volun-
tarily through EPGE. This might be due to the fact that the former
does not address the core issue of animal experiments representing a
conflict situation per se. It is evident that these two guidelines have
different starting points in this respect. However, given the overarching aim of the Basel Declaration to create public trust and freedom
of research, it would have been relevant also to consider the ethical
dilemma of research with animals.

5.5.2 *Specific Guidelines on Good Practice in Research with Animals*

Guidelines for scientific research mean to improve the quality of science by helping researchers to better designed and performed experiments. When it comes to the use of animals in biomedical research,
preoccupations about how results translate from preclinical studies
with animals to clinical studies with humans has been a major driver to
develop guidelines for animal experiments.

Several guidelines have been developed for different areas of
research with the central aim of improving quality of studies, and
we here present seven such guidelines from a range of disciplines.
In these guidelines several issues of study design, characteristics of
animal models, techniques of assessment and translational concerns
are addressed and discussed, and to some extent also issues related
to the ethical use of animals and the importance of how to minimize
animal suffering and pain (see Table 5.2).

Finally, the perhaps best-known guidelines focus on how animal experiments are reported rather than how they are executed.
The lack of information in published articles can also negatively
affect the quality of science, because poorly reported studies cannot

Table 5.2 *Overview of guidelines for animal research*

	ALS (The Basel (Ludolph et al., 2010))	Animal behaviour (Anonymous, 1997)	Cancer (Workman et al., 2010)	Myasthenia Gravis (Phillips et al., 2015)	Veterinary oncology (Webster et al., 2011)	Rett syndrome (Katz et al., 2012)	Stroke (Fisher et al., 2009)
Experimental animals							
Genetic background	•						
Sex	•		•	•	•	•	•
Experimental procedures							
Phenotype of disease progression	•		•	•	•	•	•
Outcome measures	•		•	•	•	•	•
Statistical analysis	•		•	•	•	•	
Experimental design							
Pilot studies	•	•	•				
Sample size	•	•	•	•	•	•	•
Randomization and/ or blinding				•	•	•	•
Inclusion/exclusion criteria						•	•

	1	2	3	4	5	6	7
Validity and replication							
External validity of data		•	•	•			•
Replication and reproducibility	•	•	•				•
Efficacy of treatment	•				•		•
Animal care and 3Rs							
Recommendations and legislation		•		•	•	•	
Harms versus benefits				•	•	•	
Refinement of procedures				•	•	•	
Housing and husbandry					•	•	
Training				•		•	

Source: Original table by Joana Fernandes.

be correctly evaluated and interpreted or reproduced in independent laboratories. A team of scientists developed the ARRIVE guidelines (Kilkenny *et al.*, 2010), aiming to improve completeness of information in articles, that consequently will improve the quality of scientific research in a very broad range of areas. This document has been adopted by several scientific journals since it was published in 2010.

QUESTIONS FOR DISCUSSION AND REFLECTION

1. Describe the main content of the legislation on the use of animals in research in the country where you perform research.
2. In relation to your own research or the research you are involved in, which aspects of legislation are relevant in an ethics review? Would another legislation, e.g. the European Directive (2010/63/EU) or North American guidelines, point at other aspects?
3. Different ethical issues are evoked depending on focus, e.g. experimental animals or experimental procedures etc. (left column in Table 5.2). Mention the three types of issues covered in Table 5.2 you consider are the most relevant (a) for your research and (b) in general, and explain your answers.
4. What arguments for and against regulation of the use of animals in research are the most convincing? What speaks in favour of legislation and voluntary guidelines, respectively?

REFERENCES

AAALAC (American Association for the Assessment and Accreditation of Laboratory of Animal Care). (2015). Rules of accreditation (Section 1. Definition. Laboratory Animals). www.aaalac.org/accreditation/rules.cfm (accessed 12 December 2016).

Abbott, A. (2010). Lab-animal battle reaches truce. *Nature News*, 464: 964.

Alexius Borgström, K. (2009). *Djuren, läkarna och lagen: en rättslig studie om djurförsöksetik*. Uppsala: Justus förlag.

Animal Procedures Committee (APC). (2003). Review of Cost-Benefit Assessment in the Use of Animals in Research. Report of the Cost-Benefit Working Group of the Animal Procedures Committee. Home Office, Communication Directorate, London.

Anonymous. (1997). Guidelines for the treatment of animals in behavioural research and teaching. *Animal Behaviour*, 53: 229–234.

Anonymous. (2008). Proposed reform to animal testing rules draws fire. *Nature*, 456: 152.

The Basel Declaration. (2015). http://www.basel-declaration.org (accessed 12 December 2016).

Brody, B. A. (1998). *The ethics of biomedical research: An international perspective.* Oxford: Oxford University Press.

Canadian Council on Animal Care (CCAC). (1991). CCAC policy statement on: categories of invasiveness in animal experiments. http://www.ccac.ca/en_/standards/policies/policy-categories_of_invasiveness (accessed 12 December 2016).

Canadian Council on Animal Care (CCAC). (1997). CCAC Guide to Protocol Review. http://www.ccac.ca/Documents/Standards/Guidelines/Protocol_Review.pdf (accessed 12 December 2016).

Canadian Council on Animal Care (CCAC). (2006). Terms of Reference for Animal Care Committees. http://www.ccac.ca/Documents/Standards/Policies/Terms_of_reference_for_ACC.pdf (accessed 12 December 2016).

Canadian Council on Animal Care (CCAC). (2015). Working together to enhance animal ethics and care in science. Canadian Council on Animal Care Strategic Plan, 2015–2020. http://www.ccac.ca/Documents/About/CCAC_Strategic_Plan_2015-2020.pdf (accessed 12 December 2016).

CFR (Code of Federal Regulations). (1985). Animal Welfare Act (7 U.S.C. 2131) 9 CFR, 2.31 (a) (b). https://www.nal.usda.gov/awic/animal-welfare-act (accessed 9 April 2017).

Council of Europe. (1986). European Convention for the Protection of Vertebrate Animals Used for Experimental and Other Scientific Purposes. CETS No. 123. https://www.coe.int/en/web/conventions/full-list/-/conventions/treaty/123

Dresser, R. (2001). *When science offers salvation: Patient advocacy and research ethics.* New York: Oxford University Press.

European Commission. (2014a). National Competent Authorities for the implementation of Directive 2010/63/EU on the protection of animals used for scientific purposes – A working document on the development of a common education and training framework to fulfil the requirements under the Directive. http://ec.europa.eu/environment/chemicals/lab_animals/pdf/Endorsed_E-T.pdf (accessed 12 December 2016).

European Commission. (2014b). National Competent Authorities for the Implementation of Directive 2010/63/EU on the protection of animals used for scientific purposes – A working document on Animal Welfare Bodies and National Committees to fulfil the requirements under the Directive. http://ec.europa.eu/environment/chemicals/lab_animals/pdf/endorsed_awb-nc.pdf (accessed 12 December 2016).

European Commission. (2015). Animals used for scientific purposes. http:// ec.europa.eu/environment/chemicals/lab_animals/home_en.htm (accessed 12 December 2016).

European Parliament Legislative Observatory. (2010). Protection of animals used for scientific purposes. http://www.europarl.europa.eu/oeil/popups/ficheprocedure .do?lang=en&reference=2008/0211(COD) (accessed 12 December 2016).

European Union Reference Laboratory for Alternatives to Animal Testing (EURL ECVAM). (2015). https://eurl-ecvam.jrc.ec.europa.eu/ (accessed 12 December 2016).

Expert Working Group (EWG). (2013). Expert Working Group for Project Evaluation and Retrospective Assessment. National Competent Authorities for the implementation of Directive 2010/63/EU on the protection of animals used for scientific purposes. Working document on Project Evaluation and Retrospective Assessment. http://ec.europa.eu/environment/chemicals/lab_ animals/pdf/Endorsed_E-T.pdf (accessed 12 December 2016).

Federation of Animal Science Societies (FASS). (2010). The guide for the care and use of agricultural animals in research and teaching. https://www.aaalac.org/ about/Ag_Guide_3rd_ed.pdf https://www.aaalac.org/about/Ag_Guide_3rd_ ed.pdf (accessed 9 April 2017).

Federation of European Laboratory Animal Science Associations (FELASA). (2007). Outline for the revision of Directive 86/609/EEC. http://www.felasa.eu/pol- icy-documents/outline-for-the-revision-of-directive-86-609-eec (accessed 12 December 2016).

Fisher, M., Feuerstein, G., Howells, D. W., Hurn, P. D., Kent, T. A., Savitz, S. I., and Lo, E. H. (2009). Update of the stroke therapy academic industry round- table preclinical recommendations. Stroke: A Journal of Cerebral Circulation, 40(6): 2244–2250.

Government of New Zealand. (1999). Animal Welfare Act http://www.legislation .govt.nz/act/public/1999/0142/latest/DLM49664.html (accessed 12 December 2016).

Government of Uruguay. (2009). Ley n°18.611. Utilización de Animales en Actividades de Experimentación, Docencia e Investigación Científica 2009. http://www.iibce.edu.uy/ETICA/ley-18611-oct-2-2009.pdf (accessed 12 December 2016).

Guidelines for the Use of Animals. (1997). Guidelines for the treatment of animals in behavioural research and teaching. *Animal Behaviour*, 53: 229–234.

Guillén, J. (2014). *Laboratory animals: Regulations and recommendations for glo- bal collaborative research.* Cambridge: Academic Press.

Hagelin, J., Hau, J. & Carlsson, H. E. (2003). The refining influence of ethics committees on animal experimentation in Sweden. *Laboratory Animals*, 37: 10–18.

Hamm, T. E., Dell, R. B. & van Sluyters. R. C. (1995). Laboratory animal care policies and regulations: United States. *ILAR Journal*, 37: 75–78.

Hau, J., Carlsson, H. E. & Hagelin, J. (2001). Animal research: Ethics committees have influenced animal experiments in Sweden. *BMJ*, 322: 1604.

Home Office. (1986). *Animals (Scientific Procedures) Act 1986 (Chapter 14)*. London: The Stationery Office.

Ideland, M. (2009). Different views on ethics: How animal ethics is situated in a committee culture. *Journal of Medical Ethics*, 35: 258–261.

Japan Science Council. (2006). Guidelines for Proper Conduct of Animal Experiments. http://www.scj.go.jp/en/animal/

Jennings, M. & Silcock, S. (1995). Benefits, necessity and justification in animal research. *Alternatives to Laboratory Animals*, 23: 828–836.

Katz, D. M., Berger-Sweeney, J. E., Eubanks, J. H., Justice, M. J., Neul, J. L., Pozzo-Miller, L., Blue, M. E. … Zoghbi, H. Y. & Mamounas, L.A. (2012). Preclinical research in Rett syndrome: Setting the foundation for translational success. *Disease Models & Mechanisms*, 5: 733–745.

Kilkenny, C., Browne, W. J., Cuthill, I. C., Emerson, M. & Altman, D. G. (2010). Improving bioscience research reporting: The ARRIVE guidelines for reporting animal research. *PLoS Biology*, 8: e1000412.

Laber, K. Newcomer, C. E. Decelle, T. Everitt, J. I. Guillén, J. & Brønstad, A. (2016). Recommendations for addressing harm-benefit analysis and implementation in ethical evaluation – Report from the AALAS-FELASA working group on harm-benefit analysis – part 2. *Laboratory Animals*, 50: 21–42.

Linzay, A. (1995). *Animal theology*. Urbana: University of Illinois Press.

Ludolph, A. C., Bendotti, C., Blaugrund, E., Chio, A., Greensmith, L., Loeffler, J. P., Mead, R. … Vieira, F. & von Horsten, S. (2010). Guidelines for preclinical animal research in ALS/MND: A consensus meeting. *Amyotrophic Lateral Sclerosis*, 11: 38–45.

Mendelsohn, E. (1987). The political anatomy of controversy in the sciences. In T. J. Engelhart & A. Caplan (eds.), *Scientific controversies: Case studies in the resolution and closure of disputes in science and technology*. Cambridge: Cambridge University Press, pp. 93–124.

Messerli – Research Institute. (2012). University of Veterinary Medicine Vienna. Developing a methodology to evaluate animal experiments. http://www.vetmeduni.ac.at/en/messerli/science/ethik/projects/methodology-for-the-evaluation-of-animal-experiments/ (accessed 30 November 2014).

Ministry of Agriculture Food and Rural Affairs (South Korea). (1991) Animal Protecting Act. (revised 2008).

Ministry of Environment and Forest I. (1960). The Prevention of Cruelty to Animals Act. No. 59 of 1960. http://www.awbi.org/awbi-pdf/Act%20&%20 Rules%20-%20English.pdf

Ministry of Environment and Forest I. (1998a). S.O.732 (E), [26/8/1998] – The Experiments on Animals (Controls and Supervision) (Amendment) Rules. http://envfor.nic.in/legis/awbi/awbi04.html (accessed 12 December 2016).

Ministry of Environment and Forest I. (1998b). S.O.1074, [15/12/1998] – The Breeding of and Experiments on Animals (Control and Supervision) Rules. http://envfor.nic.in/legis/awbi/awbi10.html (accessed 12 December 2016).

Ministry of Environment and Forest I (2001) S.O.134 (E), [15/2/2001] – The Breeding of and Experiments on animals (Control and Supervision) Amendment Rules. http://envfor.nic.in/legis/awbi/awbi11.html (accessed 12 December 2016).

Ministry of Science and Technology (MOST), China. (2006). Guidelines of humane treatment of laboratory animals. http://www.most.gov.cn/fggw/zfwj/ zfwj2006/200609/t20060930_54389.htm

Monamy, V. (2009). *Animal experimentation: A guide to the issues.* Cambridge: Cambridge University Press.

National Health and Medical Research Council (NHMRC). (2013). Australian Code of Practice for the Care and Use of Animals for Scientific Purposes, 8th ed. http://www.nhmrc.gov.au/guidelines/publications/ea28 (accessed 12 December 2016).

National Research Council (NRC). (2011). Guide for the Care and Use of Laboratory Animals: 8th edition. https://grants.nih.gov/grants/olaw/Guide-for-the-Care- and-use-of-laboratory-animals.pdf (accessed 12 December 2016).

National Science Board (NSB). (2014). Reducing investigators' administrative workload for federally funded research. https://www.nsf.gov/pubs/2014/ nsb1418/nsb1418.pdf

Office of Laboratory Animal Welfare (OLAW). (2002). *Public health service policy on humane care and use of laboratory animals.* Bethesda, MD: NIH Publication.

Olsson, I. A. S., Hansen, A. K. & Sandøe, P. (2008). Animal welfare and the refine- ment of neuroscience research methods – a case study of Huntington's disease models. *Laboratory Animals*, 42: 277–283.

Olsson, I. A. S., Silva, S. P., Townend, D. & Sandøe, P. (2016) Protecting animals and enabling research in the European Union: An overview of development and implementation of Directive 2010/63/EU. *ILAR Journal.* 57: 347–357.

Ormandy, E. H. (2012). The use of animals in research: Trends and public attitudes. Doctor of Philosophy Thesis, Faculty of Graduate Studies, Animal Science,

University of British Columbia, Vancouver, BC. http://lfs-awp.sites.olt.ubc.ca/ files/2012/11/ubc_2012_fall_ormandy_elisabeth.pdf (accessed April 9, 2017).

Ormandy, E. H., Dale, J. & Griffin, G. (2013). Use of genetically-engineered animals in science: Perspectives of Canadian animal care committee members. *Alternatives to Laboratory Animals*, 41: 1–8.

Persson, S. (2009). Etisk prövning: nästan alla djurförsök godkänns. Göteborg: TGM. http://www.djurensratt.se/sites/default/files/etiskprovning_0.pdf (accessed 12 December 2016).

Phillips, B. & Jennings, M. (2008). Home Office licence abstracts – an assessment. *Atla-Alternatives to Laboratory Animals*, 36: 465–471.

Phillips, W. D., Christadoss, P., Losen, M., Punga, A. R., Shigemoto, K., Verschuuren, J. & Vincent, A. (2015). Guidelines for pre-clinical animal and cellular models of MuSK-myasthenia gravis. *Experimental Neurology*, 270: 29–40.

Plous, S. & Herzog, H. (2001). Reliability of protocol reviews for animal research. *Science*, 293: 608–609.

Preece, R. (2002). *Awe for the tiger, love for the lamb: A chronicle of sensibility to animals*. Vancouver: UBC Press.

Presidência da República CC. (2008). Presidência da República CC, Subchefia para Assuntos Jurídicos, Brazil. Lei n° 11.794 de 8 de Outubro, 2008 ('Arouca Law'). http://www.planalto.gov.br/ccivil_03/_ato2007-2010/2008/lei/l11794.htm (accessed 12 December 2016).

Ringblom, J., Törnqvist, E., Hansson, S. O., Rudén, C. & Öberg, M. (2017). Assigning ethical weights to clinical signs observed during toxicity testing. *ALTEX*, 34: 148–156.

Röcklinsberg, H. (2015). Lay persons involvement and public interest. Ethical assessment in animal ethics committees in Sweden. The Swedish Transition Process of the EU Directive 2010/ 63/ EU with regard to Harm- Benefit Analysis in Animal Ethics Committees. *ALTEX Proceedings*, 4(1): 45–48.

Ruhdel, I., Maisack, C. & Wagner, K. (2014). German animal welfare act in breach with Directive 2010/63/EU. *ALTEX*, 31: 219–222. doi: http://dx.doi.org/ 10.14573/altex.1404011

Russell, W. & Burch, R. (1959). *The principles of humane experimental technique*. London: Methuen & Co. Ltd.

Schiermeier, Q. (2008). German authority halts primate work. *Nature*, 455: 1159.

Schuppli, C. A. (2011). Decisions about the use of animals in research: Ethical reflection by Animal ethics committee members. *Anthrozoös*, 24: 409–425.

Schuppli, C. A. & Fraser, D. (2005). The interpretation and application of the three Rs by animal ethics committee members. *Alternatives to Laboratory Animals*, 33: 1–14.

Schuppli, C. A. & Fraser, G. (2007). Factors influencing the effectiveness of research ethics committees. *Journal of Medical Ethics*, 33: 294–301.

Schuppli, C. A., Fraser, D. & McDonald, M. (2004). Expanding the three Rs to meet new challenges in humane animal experimentation. *Alternatives to Laboratory Animals*, 32: 525–532.

Secretaría de Agricultura. (2001). Secretaría de Agricultura G, Desarrollo Rural, Pesca y Alimentación, Mexico. NOM-062-ZOO-1999. Especificaciones Técnicas para la Producción, Cuidado y Uso de Animales de Laboratorio. Diario Oficial de la Federación 22 de agosto de 2001. http://www.fmvz.unam.mx/fmvz/principal/archivos/062ZOO.PDF (accessed 12 December 2016).

Smith, J., van den Broek, F., Martorell, J. C., Hackbarth, H., Ruksenas, O. & Zeller, W. (2007). Principles and practice in ethical review of animal experiments across Europe: Summary of the report of a FELASA working group on ethical evaluation of animal experiments. *Laboratory Animals*, 41: 143–160.

Vasbinder, M. A., Hawk, C. T. & Bennett, B. T. (2014). Regulations, policies, and guidelines impacting laboratory animal welfare. In K. Bayne & P. V. Turner (eds.), *Laboratory animal welfare* (pp. 17–28). Waltham, MA: Elsevier Inc.

Vieira de Castro, A. C. & Olsson, I. A. (2015). Does the goal justify the methods? Harm and benefit in neuroscience research using animals. *Current Topics in Behavioral Neurosciences*, 19: 47–78.

Walters, K. S. & Portmess, L. (1999). *Ethical vegetarianism: From Pythagoras to Peter Singer*. Albany: SUNY Press.

Webster, J. D., Dennis, M. M., Dervisis, N., Heller, J., Bacon, N. J., Bergman, P. J., Bienzle, D. ... Yager, J. & Kiupel, M. (2011). Recommended guidelines for the conduct and evaluation of prognostic studies in veterinary oncology. *Veterinary Pathology*, 48: 7–18.

Workman, P., Aboagye, E. O., Balkwill, F., Balmain, A., Bruder, G., Chaplin, D. J., Double, J. A. ... Wedge, S. R. & Eccles, S. A. (2010). Guidelines for the welfare and use of animals in cancer research. *British Journal of Cancer*, 102: 1555–1577.

6   Public Involvement: How and Why?

With Jesper Lassen and Thomas Bøker Lund
(Sections 6.1 and 6.2); Karin Gabrielsson
Morton and Mats Sjöqvist (Section 6.3);
and Franck L. B. Meijboom (Section 6.4)

This chapter focuses on public involvement in animal-based research. As discussed in the previous chapter, laypersons are within some legislative frameworks involved in the actual project evaluation through participation in animal ethics committees, while this is not the case within other frameworks. The general public may involve itself, or be asked to engage in judgement of ethical issues in research on animals in other forms like expressing their opinion on surveys or participating in workshops or debates.

Since understanding of different viewpoints form our perspective and facilitates a nuanced discussion, it is relevant for researchers to know what concerns society in general holds about animal use in research. Here we wish to stress the pragmatic point that if there is too large a distance between public perceptions of if and when animal research can be justified and the practice of the research community, criticism of animal research in general will probably grow. As a consequence, even research that the majority initially found acceptable might be difficult to find support for. It is thus both in the interest of researchers and the general public to have an open and transparent dialogue on the circumstances of animal research and on what is necessary to justify it. Whether or not a certain opinion held by the general public is justified is a topic for a separate discussion and is not covered in this chapter.

In Section 6.1 we elaborate on different reasons for involving the general public; in Section 6.2 we present some studies on attitudes about using animals in research; whereas Section 6.3 presents a discussion of the relation between funding and public involvement. Finally, in Section 6.4 we elaborate on democratic aspects of animal ethics committees, and on how public interest can be taken into account.

6.1 WHY INVOLVE PEOPLE IN DECISIONS OVER THE USE OF ANIMALS IN RESEARCH?

Historically, arrangements aimed at involving the public in political decision-making beyond simply voting dates back to the 1930s. This kind of lay participation has taken place within different policy areas such as societal planning, domestic politics and in the most recent decades in relation to science and technology, including issues related to the use of laboratory animals. On the one hand, lay participation has been justified simply as a fundamental feature of democracy. On the other hand, a more pragmatic line of thought exists, stressing the need of participatory arrangements as necessary means to solve anticipated or existing social controversies (see e.g. Nielsen *et al.*, 2007; Rowe and Frewer, 2000; van Asselt Marjolein and Rijkens-Klomp, 2002). It should be noted that there is a great variation among political cultures as to what extent participation beyond voting is acknowledged as a legitimate activity. Some countries, such as the Scandinavian ones, have a more participatory political culture favouring public involvement, while other countries, such as France, have a more technocratic political culture in which involvement primarily is secured by means of the representative democracy (Nielsen *et al.*, 2004).

The popularity of public involvement that can be witnessed in many western countries during the past five decades can largely be ascribed to growing awareness of the side effects of industrialization that emerged in the 1960s. Thus, the emerging critique of not only industrial but also agricultural production raised concerns among the public that sometimes developed into controversies (Harrison, 1964; Vapnek and Chapman, 2010). With regard to animals this has been seen in relation for example the cloning of animals, fur production and the use of animals for research purposes. Such controversies, and in some cases even the fear of a controversy, has called for a more proactive approach to socially negotiate technologies and their regulation by involving the public more than just through representative democracy. Thus participatory methods have been advanced with the idea that a timely involvement of the public would ensure that the development would be seen as more acceptable or legitimate by the general public.

6.1.1 *Ways of Involving the Public*

There has been a change in the understanding of how involvement could contribute to greater public acceptance. Up to the 1970s, the dominating perception was more or less that decisions on technologies should be left to the experts, and public involvement was perceived as enlightening non-experts. Within this understanding, the basic idea was that resistance to science and technology can be explained by lacking knowledge. Thus technological development was seen as a given fact, and involvement took the shape of one-way communication often through information campaigns or public meetings. As a reaction, a different approach emerged during the late 1970s and 1980s, promoting the idea that technologies are to a large extent shaped by social actors. According to this understanding, decisions about technologies – including those that involve animals in one way or the other – should involve the public as well as other interested parties in a dialogue. In this kind of dialogue, ideally the participatory arrangements should not only ensure the delivery of information to the public but also make sure public concerns are taken into consideration and have a real chance to influence guidelines and regulation of technologies.

It is the latter approach that today most often is associated with public involvement – largely thanks to the emergence of Boards of Technology or similar institutions having as their responsibility to develop participatory methods and ensure public involvement in discussions of pending and potential technologies. When looking into the toolbox of participatory methods, it is noticeable that the different methods vary greatly when it comes to degree of involvement. See Table 6.1 for an overview of methods to involve the public.

At one end we find methods where experts gather information about public concerns, interests or needs using qualitative or quantitative research methods. These are by far the most common means of involvement, and typical examples include the use of focus group interviews or surveys to get a better understanding of how the general public perceives a new technology or practice – in this case the use of animals in research. Often the research is commissioned by companies using animals or public authorities responsible for development of the regulation of research animals.

At the other end of the scale are methods in which participation is more genuinely a two-way process. Here decision-makers and the general public are engaged in a dialogue with the potential to affect both parties through methods such as consensus conferences and citizen juries. The understanding of involvement at this end of the scale is often described as a deliberation among the affected parties. Such interactive involvement processes were, however, mainly used in the 1990s, and are today replaced by activities a bit lower on the ladder of participation. Thus, in the area of research animals, relatively cheaper methods such as focus groups and surveys are the most common means of public involvement.

6.1.2 *Involvement in Animal Research Is Low in the General Public*

Historically animal research has caught considerable attention in the media because of the moral outrage that is triggered by textual and especially visual presentation of maltreatment of animals during experimentation. In this respect, it is likely that most lay people across nations have been confronted with the animal research issue.

Table 6.1 *An overview of common means of public involvement.*

Arrangement	Description
Consensus Conference	In the consensus conferences in the shape of the so-called Danish model the basic idea is to give lay people a voice in the political processes by selecting a panel of lay people (12–15 persons) who are given the power to set the agenda in a pending controversy. Thus the lay panel formulates the questions that need to be answered by experts. At the end of the conference the lay panel produces a document presenting their consensus on the issue at hand.
Future Workshop	In a future workshop (lay) participants are guided through a structured debate in three phases. First, participants are allowed to criticize anything related to the issue, without being contradicted. Second, visions about the issue in question are formulated without paying respect to barriers; and third, strategies to realize the visions are discussed.
Delphi Studies/ Technology Foresight	Methods where a large number of stakeholder representatives are invited to, through a survey, give their opinion about the future. Panels with representatives from user groups are appointed and meet at a number of workshops, and finally all gather to draw conclusions and formulate recommendations.
Public representation in decision fora	Public representatives are designated as members in committees or boards that handle e.g. legislative decision, allocation of resources or where future policies are decided upon.
Focus Groups	A qualitative interview format where a small group (typically 5–12) is gathered and guided through a structured discussion. The interviews are analysed by social scientists.

(continued)

Table 6.1 *(continued)*

Arrangement	Description
Surveys	A quantitative method where respondents are contacted by phone, mail, internet or personally and asked to fill out a questionnaire. The data are subsequently analysed by social scientists/ statisticians.
Public Consultation/ Citizen Consultation	A widespread and common means of participation, where the public is invited to participate in the decision-making process, either at public meetings or through a call for (written) comments.
Referendum	Popular vote on a specific issue, including all affected citizens in a region or nation. Particularly used in Switzerland.
Citizen Initiatives	In the EU, the Treaty of Lisbon opens for an issue to be discussed in the European Parliament if signed by 1 million citizens.

Source: Adapted from Nielsen et al (2004).

Media attention does not, however, necessarily reflect the level of public engagement with the topic. Unfortunately, there is little direct research into how the public engage in animal research, and some of it is quite dated. However, interpretations offered from available data suggest that the general public's involvement in this type of animal use is quite modest. A significant proportion of the public is not interested and involved in political issues at all, and amongst those that do find politics and political issues relevant, the use of animals is not a particularly salient topic.

This might reflect a generally low public interest in the use of animals in general, but there might also be a difference between a general interest in politics on the one hand and in animals on the other, as well as differences related to forms of animal use and between regions. Polls from the United States in the late 1980s showed treatment of animal to be ranked as the least important of 12 issues facing the country (Herzog *et al.*, 2001). More recently, only 13% of the Danish public mentioned animal welfare as one of the three most important issues when choosing a political party to vote for at the national election. Specifically with respect to animal research, only 9% of Danes in 2011 felt that they are engaged in animal research and 10% stated that they often discuss animal research with friends and family (Lund, 2011). According to the Eurobarometer 2016 (European Commission, 2016) where informants were not asked to rank issues, but merely to agree or disagree to certain statements, a majority (94%) of European citizens answer they consider farm animal welfare important, 82% think farm animal welfare should be better protected, whereas 74% agree the welfare of companion animals should be better protected. Although not directly comparable with regard to methodology, according to a 2014 UK study, 7–8% of the UK public report to know a great deal or a fair amount with respect to 3R-relevant questions and 6% knew of the National Centre for the 3Rs. This concerns a more specific field of knowledge than concern for animal welfare in general, but still the level can be regarded as low (Leaman *et al.*, 2014).

The reason for the low public interest is probably explained by the busy everyday lives that ordinary people have. There is not much time to devote to politics or wider societal issues in general (Herzog *et al.*, 2001). In the face of this time constraint, political issues that appear close or important in everyday life, whether it is taxation, economics, health care or access to public services, are assigned higher priority. The welfare of animals appears simply to be outcompeted by other political topics, despite the fact that a large majority agree that they are concerned about animals' welfare in general, including in animal research.

In food ethics a process known as willed blindness exists, describing how people officially argue for animal welfare but without being prepared to take steps needed to improve production forms. It is suggested that this is possible thanks to a tacit agreement between producer and consumer not to mention issues related to impaired animal welfare, threats to the environment or lack of social fairness, as this would call for being prepared to pay for a change in production systems as well as purchase behaviour (Gjerris, 2015). Furthermore, consumers develop strategies of moral disengagement from animals (Graça *et al.*, 2014). Translated to animal research, willed blindness highlights a potential agreement between citizens, (potential) patients, representatives from the pharmaceutical industry and researchers not to debate animal welfare, and even less animal ethics or use of animals in research as such, as that would call for scrutiny of the risk of undue suffering, poor research results, as well as the perceived right to development of new treatment methods and drugs.

6.1.3 *Political Activity in Engaged Public Subgroups*

Due to the low interest level in the European populations as such, it is not to be expected that the large public majority will embark on political activity addressing animal research or take animal research into consideration in e.g. electoral voting. Nevertheless, in some public subgroups there are many political activities in relation to animal issues in general and research animals especially. A wide range of organizations engage in the animal experimentation issue, whereof some aim at improving the situation for animals (e.g. Royal Society for the Prevention of Cruelty to Animals, RSPCA) and some at a total ban of use of animals in research (e.g. People for the Ethical Treatment of Animals, PETA). They may perform surveys or polls to investigate public views, but in general base their activities on being representative of their members, and work by lobby and campaigns to evoke political as well as public interest. Hence the public involvement is channelled through these organizations rather than asked for by decision-makers. A new kind of public involvement in animal research of special interest here is a recent citizen incentive in the EU, called Stop Vivisection.

The European Citizens' Initiative (ECI) aims at increasing direct democracy in the European Union (European Commission, 2015a).

By collecting signatures from at least one million EU citizens from seven member states EU citizens can request the Commission to take legal action. This gives citizens the same right to request the Commission to initiate a legislative proposal as the European Parliament and Council. Since its launch in May 2012, only three have gathered the minimum number of signatures to be considered by the Commission. One of the three successful ECIs concerns animal experimentation. Stop Vivisection was launched in 2013 to 'urge the European Commission to abrogate directive 2010(63/EU) on the protection of animals used for scientific purposes and to present a new proposal that does away with animal experimentation and instead makes compulsory the use – in biomedical and toxicological research – of data directly relevant for the human species' (Stop Vivisection, 2015). In June 2015, the response from The European Commission was published: it agrees that the use of animals in research should be phased out. However, as this aim is expressed in the recently implemented directive and animal-based research is still needed, no alternative legislation will replace it at this moment (European Commission, 2015b). This ECI collected signatories from many European countries, with a high proportion from Italy. One can expect that these persons are engaged in the issue and have a different view on animal research than less engaged citizens do.

6.2 STUDIES OF ATTITUDES TO ANIMAL RESEARCH

It is sometimes argued that disapproval is based on lack of information or on ideology (Rollin, 2006), and that since the general public lacks interest in animal research, one could assume that people do not really have a well-formed attitude about it and cannot deliberate meaningfully on the topic. However, empirical studies require in-depth investigations of public attitude formation, and there are only a few countries where the data is complete enough to ascertain this: the United Kingdom and Denmark (see additional discussion later in the chapter). The findings from both countries show very clearly that lay people in fact are very capable of forming attitudes to animal research. Thus, in a Danish qualitative study the participants easily deliberated on the topic and developed reasoned attitudes (Lund *et al.*, 2012), and studies in the United Kingdom show comparable results (Aldhous *et al.*, 1999). Danish studies further showed that 21% of disapprovers report they are involved in the debate, compared to 5.5% of the remaining respondents (Lund *et al.*, 2012; 2014). Further, these studies show that 22% of disapprovers report that they often talk with friends/relatives about animal research, compared to 7% of approvers, and that disapprovers have higher certainty of attitudes (they are not likely to change opinion).

A thorough mapping of a country's attitude to animal research must as a minimum seek to measure the prevalence of three fundamentally different attitude stances. Research in the United Kingdom (Corrado *et al.*, 2010) and Denmark (Lund *et al.*, 2014) points at three groups differing in their level of acceptance: from 'objectors'/ 'disapprovers' to conditional 'acceptors'/'reserved' to 'unconditional acceptors'/'approvers'. While there are differences between the methodologies of these two studies, it is clear from both of them that objectors/disapprovers constitute a minority of the respective publics. By definition, then, a public majority does not reject this sort of animal use. Whether this is the case in other countries is an open question, until elaborate inquiries have been made.

It is also clear that among the large group who do not reject animal experimentation per se, such experimentation can only be accepted under certain conditions. More specifically, it is a proviso that there are clear human gains from the research and that animals will not suffer strongly. In practice this means that people embark on a refined weighting of the research aim against animal welfare in concrete research designs. Thus, public approval rates of specific research designs vary considerably depending on research aim, suffering to the animals, and animal species (Aldhous *et al.*, 1999; Lund *et al.*, 2014).

The ongoing Eurobarometer surveys have multiple times included question items regarding support for animal research. This has the clear advantage of enabling country comparisons and detecting changes over time, and it has been showed that public acceptance of animal research across European countries was about 45% in 2001, which slightly decreased to 43% by 2005 (von Roten (2009). Unfortunately, the Eurobarometer question items are not well equipped to distinguish attitudinal differences that are likely to be in play in most nation states (Lund *et al.*, 2014).

Hence, citizens engaged in political activities related to animals are often opposed to animal research or at least to an unconditional and uncritical acceptance of such research. These differences in levels of engagement could be seen as a mirror – when it comes to engaged lay people – of a link between on the one hand knowledge about research results and practices and on the other disapproval based on a fundamental value of respect for individual animal welfare, or animal's rights to life, which differs from the view of citizens approving animal research, much in line with researchers themselves.

6.2.1 *Changes in Policy: Is the Public Pushing?*

As shown in the preceding sections, there have recently been considerable citizen initiatives to phase out or at least reduce animal experimentation in the EU. In line with the regulation of the Directive 2010/63, centres have also been established to promote the use of non-animal alternatives, e.g. EURL-ECVAM (European Union Reference Laboratory for Alternatives to Animal Testing), and breeders, suppliers and research institutes are required to establish an animal welfare body to facilitate implementation of 3R (preamble 31). Considering the lack of involvement among the general public, one can raise the question whether and how citizens have pushed in this direction. However, the process formulating the Directive was lengthy, and although only on a political level, aimed at establishing a harmonized legislation on a level possible to implement in all member states (see also Chapter 5).

While we can only speculate about this, it is likely that the public in fact has played a part in establishment of stricter regulation regarding animal research. This is not due to e.g. consensus conferences, workshops, public consultations (Table 6.1), which to our knowledge not have been drafted with respect to animal research. Instead, the public has probably played a role in two different ways. First, since the 1960s, the general concern for animal welfare has steadily increased in European countries (Sandøe and Christiansen, 2013). This development is parallel to increased industrialization of housing, transport and slaughter of farm animals, and concerns are reflected in increased legislation related to animal protection/welfare in general and in specific domains of use. In this respect 'indirect' pressure from a more concerned public can have pushed forward. The second and probably more important way in which members of the public have pushed is through the demonstrations and activism that has occurred primarily in the United Kingdom. Already in the early 1970s, UK animal rights activists attacked laboratories with animal facilities, and there are numerous accounts of personal threats against animal experimenters. Therefore, especially in the United Kingdom there has been focus on the ethical basis of animal research. Indeed, the United Kingdom was the first nation to decide on a phasing out of cosmetics testing. This decision later spread out to all the other EU member states.

6.2.2 *Dialogue with the Public*

Involvement of the public in the debate must not be seen by the research community only as a chance to convince the public about the necessity of animal use in medical research, but may possibly also be taken as an opportunity to listen to other views on the matter. Interaction with citizens' perspectives could be regarded part of researchers' task to disseminate research and also potentially increase mutual understanding of what is regarded ethically relevant from different value perspectives. Whether information about research leads to increased or decreased acceptance is an open question, though. Entering the dialogue with this in mind, the goal of the dialogue can be to create a socially robust research practice rather than increase possibilities of doing research as much as possible.

One example of attempts to increase transparency is the yearly meetings arranged by the Swedish Research Council for stakeholders in animal research, including e.g. patient groups, animal welfare organizations and the general public. Themes cover updates on legislation, animal-based research focussing on recent results with regard and alternative and refined methods. On the internationally held World Day for Laboratory Animals on 24th April seminars and workshops are arranged by animal welfare organizations in many countries inviting researchers to present their research – often with focus on the 3Rs – for interested citizens. On a legal level, the Directive 2010/63/EU requires a so-called non-technical summary describing the aim of study and the harm caused in an accurate way. It should be publicly available in order to increase transparency. In the Netherlands, for instance, these summaries are made public on the website of the central ethical committee, and in accordance with the Directive, any citizen may request the documents that underlie the license.

6.3   PUBLIC FUNDING OF ANIMAL RESEARCH: THE ROLE OF FUNDING ACTORS

Society has a legitimate interest in how animal research is conducted, not only because animal welfare is an issue of societal relevance but also because the public pays for this research. Almost all medical research outside industry is publicly funded, either directly through taxes or through private research funds, which in turn are funded by donations and legacies from the public.

As discussed in the previous section, changes in policy are likely to reflect public pressure to reduce the use of animals for research and testing. The recitals of the European Directive 2010/63/EU, i. e. the part of the directive which lays down the reasons for the legal act, clearly express a desire to work towards a stronger implementation of the 3Rs. For example, Recital 10 states that

> this Directive represents an important step towards achieving the final goal of full replacement of procedures on live animals for

scientific and educational purposes as soon as it is scientifically possible to do so. To that end, it seeks to facilitate and promote the advancement of alternative approaches. It also seeks to ensure a high level of protection for animals that still need to be used in procedures. This Directive should be reviewed regularly in light of evolving science and animal-protection measures.

This points to a role of the public funding bodies in not accepting status quo in terms of animal use but to promote the 3Rs in different ways, including contributing to a culture of care when animals are actually used. Public funding bodies may also find a role in establishing a more direct dialogue with the public over research with animals.

6.3.1 Promoting the 3Rs

Funding agencies can engage in promoting the 3Rs in several ways. They can provide dedicated funding for research into replacement, refinement and/or reduction, they can incorporate research animal ethics and the 3Rs in the review of applications and they can incorporate demands for compliance into the management of funding.

In 2005, Kleveland listed 11 European countries providing specific funding for 3Rs research, including governmental as well as other funding agencies (Kleveland, 2005). Of these, the UK government's National Centre for the 3Rs (NC3Rs) is by far the largest contributor, in 2014 distributing more than 5 million GBP through project grants, strategic awards and student/research fellowships (NC3Rs, 2014). On the European level, funding has above all been provided for replacement alternatives in drug development, chemical toxicity and ecotoxicology and product safety assessment (AXLR8, 2015).

In Britain, NC3Rs have recently, in collaboration with a number of funding bodies, compiled a guidance document for guiding both funding bodies and researchers entitled: 'Responsibility in the use of animals in bioscience research. Expectations of the major research councils and charitable funding bodies' (NC3Rs, 2015). It lists some basic requirements that need to be fulfilled for funding to be granted, including that the research comply with legal provisions and relevant codes and guidelines, and that procedures and euthanasia are only performed by trained/licensed staff. The guidelines go on to state that researchers, veterinary and animal care staff need to adopt a culture of care with regard to the animals and keep updated on the development of good practices and advances in the 3Rs (see also Chapter 3). Further, the key role of ethics committees in ensuring high standards is highlighted.

The guidelines also require peer review of research applications to assess whether the research question could be addressed without the use of animals, and if the number of animals and the experimental design are optimal. All steps should be taken to minimize any pain, suffering, distress, lasting harm as well as other adverse effects arising from the scientific procedures, housing, husbandry and any travel, throughout the life of the animal. It is made clear in the guidance document that if the applicant does not address these points, the funding bodies are likely to reject the application. In the United Kingdom, the NC3Rs also provide 3Rs peer review and advice service to several major funding bodies within the country.

Funding agencies can also play an active role in ensuring compliance with legal demands. For example, the national research funding agency in Portugal, Fundação para a Ciência e a Tecnologia (FCT), will only release moneys for funded projects after the principal investigator has shown proof that they have institutional and personal licenses and have applied for a project license for the research in question (Anna Olsson, personal communication).

As Figure 6.1 illustrates, these different measures correspond to different hierarchical levels of promoting the 3Rs:

a) By demanding that grant holders comply with legislation, the funding agencies contribute to the enforcement of current minimum standards.
b) By providing guidance on higher standards researchers are given an incentive to improve welfare above legislation.

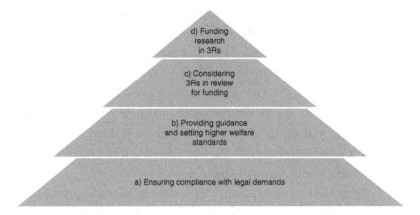

FIGURE 6.1 Different measures correspond to different hierarchical levels of promoting the 3Rs.
Source: Original figure by Röcklinsberg, Gjerris and Olsson.

c) By considering the 3Rs in funding applications, funding bodies contribute to research which takes the 3Rs seriously.

d) By providing funding for 3R research funding bodies contribute to the development of new ways of replacing, reducing and refining the use of animals in research.

6.4 THE PUBLIC OPINION AND THE ROLE OF ANIMAL ETHICS COMMITTEES

Considering the content of public debates on use of animals in research it is important to note that they may take many forms. Sometimes they focus on the general question of the availability of alternatives for use of animal. In other cases a specific research forms the start of a public debate, such as the use of dogs for cardiovascular disease research. One way to address the concerns in society is the use of ethical committees. This section aims to discuss three related questions in the view of public involvement: What role does AECs play? What role should they play? And what is the position of the public opinion in this context?

6.4.1 *What Role Should an Animal Ethics Committee Play in Relation to Society?*

Using animals is not just a private matter of a researcher. It is a matter of public discussion. Therefore, next to the ethical deliberation by the involved researchers, an independent and impartial ethical justification is required as a way to answer the public concerns with respect to animal research (Röcklinsberg *et al.*, 2014; Schuppli, 2011). Animal ethics committees can function as a bridge between science and society. On the one hand, the AEC has a direct link with the research field, e.g. since the assessment of research protocols requires sufficient competence in science, the composition of the AEC includes scientists. On the other hand, an AEC clearly has a public position. Their reasons for existence are the public concerns, and in order to voice these concerns in some countries non-experts are members of these committees. In this way, the ethical evaluation and authorization of a research project can be seen as a way to make the responsibility towards animals and the public operational. This position – as a bridge between the practice of science and society – enables a committee to discuss and assess animal research in a meaningful way, but also guarantee certain levels of impartiality and independence. The task of an AEC consists of the assessment of both the relevance of the aim(s) of a project and of the potential harms that are related to the project. Furthermore, the task includes an assessment of how well the 3Rs are met. In general, the legal framework in which the AEC operates prescribes that a project is ethically justified if and only if the project (a) has (public) relevance (scientific or societal), (b) this relevance can outweigh the harm to the animals, and if (c) there are no real options in terms of replacement, refinement and reduction.

6.4.2 *Can AECs Meet the Expectations?*

The animal ethics committees have a quite difficult task. They are supposed to make complex assessments of values that are either promoted and protected or may be infringed by the animal research project. Furthermore, they have to come to a moral judgement and ethical justification that either implies the approval of a project, with the implication that sentient animals will be used, or leads to a negative advice, which often equally has impact, e.g. in terms of possible frustration of health improvement or people's careers. Therefore, it should not come as a surprise that the functioning of AECs is still the subject of debate.

The criticisms are not univocal. It is possible to distinguish four types of criticism. A first type of criticism starts in the empirical claim that AECs do not make a real ethical assessment. Although they are supposed to fulfil this task, it has been claimed that AECs tend to interpret their task in a rather limited way, narrowing ethics down to an assessment of refinement and reduction only. The reasons for this reduction can be rather diverse. Vieira de Castro and Olsson (2015), for instance, accurately analyse that the exclusive attention to the 3R principles is often the result of the difficulties and lack of agreement between committees and between individual members with regard to the assessment of the aim. In these cases the focus on refinement and reduction is a way to escape the more fundamental, but difficult discussion. Another reason for the focus on the 3R discussion starts in a (mostly implicit) reference to an earlier ethical judgement. Suppose an AEC judges a project on a health-related protein as relevant and considers the use of mice as ethically justified. In a next meeting an application with the same aim is discussed, whereby the discussion tend to focus on the 3Rs rather than making a full ethical assessment again. In such cases, the discussion (implicitly) build on the ethical assessment that has been done in the first meeting. Given its public position, the AEC should make such steps as transparent and explicit as possible.

Second, criticisms are formulated with regard to the AECs because they are claimed to ignore broader moral issues, such as the general need for animal research or broader discussions on the acceptability of certain research aims. To a certain extent this is similar to the problem that such committees sometimes do not make genuine ethical assessments. However, there is more to say. Even if the AECs are genuinely committed to making an ethical assessment, they often do not spend much time on broader ethical issues (Röcklinsberg et al., 2014). Apart from problems of competence, this is the result of the position of the ethical evaluation at the end of the research chain. If a researcher can submit a project to an AEC, many moral assumptions and decisions have already been made implicitly, e.g. by funding agencies, research schools or regulatory bodies. As a consequence, the ethical evaluation by the AEC is already prestructured. Not addressing broader issues is problematic because (a) moral assumptions that are made elsewhere in the research chain are often made implicitly and (b) often these broader issues have public importance and therefore could contribute to the legitimacy of AECs in the assessment process. However, it is questionable whether an individual AEC, whose main task is to deliberate over individual applications for authorization of animal research, is the right forum for such a discussion. This discussion could instead take place in thematic meetings at research institutes as well as in open seminars arranged on a national level, through, for instance, the national committees for the protection of animals used for scientific purposes established through the EU Directive. Such a discussion on the national level would facilitate the reflection of the AECs on public concern for animals used in research (Recital 11 of the Directive) and, if found relevant, mirror this in the decision-making process.

A third type of criticism focuses on the limitation of the ethical assessment understood as a harm-benefit analysis. Already before the implementation of the Directive 2010/63/EU, the ethical assessment has often been considered as a process of weighing harms (mostly perceived in terms of discomfort to animals) and benefits. Even though it could be interpreted in a broader way, it easily can be understood as if harms and benefits are fully comparable entities on each side of the scales. Then it may be a small step to translate the harms and benefits in quantities that can be compared, exchanged or compensated. A well-known example is money: it is possible to weigh the financial costs of animal research against the estimated savings in the field of health care. This, however, is no longer an ethical review, but a financial assessment in which the broader range of moral values that underlie animal research remain unaddressed. Furthermore, one could criticize the idea of a harm-benefit analysis because of the tendency to perceive it as a welfare assessment. From a utilitarian perspective, this is not fundamental problem as long as the overall welfare is maximized. However, from other ethical perspectives, more values than welfare have to be taken in to account in an ethical assessment. Therefore, there has been proposals to broaden the moral vocabulary by including concepts such as animal integrity (Bovenkerk *et al.*, 2002; Röcklinsberg *et al.*, 2014).

Finally, some of the problems with the AECs and their work start in a more fundamental problem: the plurality in society with respect to the view on the moral position of animals. We have touched upon the problem already in the first type of criticism: the lack of agreement between committees and between individual members. However, this disagreement is not limited to the members of the committees. We can recognize this in society in general and it directly influences the public legitimacy and efficacy of the AECs. For those who do not recognize the independent moral standing of animals, the need for authorization by an independent committee is redundant. For those who consider animals as beings that have, like human, equal rights, the ethical assessment is necessary, but an evaluation of each project or study is irrelevant. From this perspective each type of animal use for research is unacceptable and never justifiable. Therefore, a committee that judges each experiment or project is unnecessary. This shows that an ethical committee is only essential and relevant from a specific public and ethical perspective and cannot answer all public concerns with regard to animal testing.

6.4.3 *How to Address Problems?*

The problems with ethical assessment and incorporating public opinions in the authorization process of animal research are not new. Consequently, many proposals have been made to address the problems. A first way to address the problems focuses on a better framework for ethical assessment. This is often translated into ethical frameworks or decision tools (Röcklinsberg, 2015). The form and function of these tools differ from model to model. At a minimum level they function as a checklist that structures the ethical evaluation process and aim to make the assessment more transparent and traceable for others. However, other tools have a more normative function and actively guide the user in the evaluation process (Schuppli, 2011). Even though each of these tools has their own weaknesses, it often helps committees to make more explicit assessments and to prevent blind spots in the evaluation.

A second way to address the mentioned problems stresses the need for the inclusion of persons from outside the research community or lay people in the ethical committees. This aims to ensure a more direct link with public opinion and to broaden the perspective of the issues that are to be discussed. For instance, killing an animal for further scientific analysis after death is considered to be a minor harm according to the legislation, but is perceived as a serious issue by the public (Meijboom and Stassen, 2016). In this context, it is important to stress that 'lay' does not imply uninformed or uneducated. It is much more a matter of being independent and unbiased.

Finally, transparency and dialogue have been put forward as essential ingredients for a well-operating ethical assessment of AECs and their public legitimacy. The ethical assessment should not be seen as a matter between scientists and AEC only. As indicated above, the ethical committee has a special position between science and society. Therefore, the evaluations by the AECs have to be transparent and communicated with the public. In practice this raises a number of questions with regard to conflicts with other ethical principles related to the privacy of researchers and the confidential character of some research. Nonetheless, a dialogue with the public is essential in two ways: to have a feeling for the plurality of moral views and arguments that can be used in the ethical deliberation and to act in an accountable way in fulfilling the task of giving authorization of animal research.

QUESTIONS FOR DISCUSSION AND REFLECTION

1. Describe at least three of the methods presented in this chapter of involving the public in decisions about the use of animals in research.

2. What arguments for and against involving the public in decisions about the use of animals in research are most convincing?

3. Describe the organization and role of animal ethics committees, or similar organs, in your country or the country where you perform your research.

4. What are the advantages and disadvantages of having an AEC composed of members from different disciplines and also lay persons from different backgrounds?

REFERENCES

Aldhous, P., Coghlan, A. & Copley, J. (1999). Animal experiments-where do you draw the line?: let the people speak. *New Scientist*, 162: 26.

AXLR8. (2015). EU-funded 3Rs research. http://www.axlr8.eu/eu-funded-3rs-research/ (accessed 7 May 2015).

Bovenkerk, B., Brom, F. W. & van Den Bergh, B. J. (2002). Brave new birds: The use of 'animal integrity' in animal ethics. *Hastings Center Report*, 32: 16–22.

Corrado, M., Rowley, H. & Evans, M. (2010). Views on animal experimentation. *Ipsos MORI*. https://www.ipsos-mori.com/Assets/Docs/Publications/sri-views-on-animal-experimentation-2010.pdf (accessed, 12 December 2016).

European Commission. (2015a). EU Citizens' Initiative. http://ec.europa.eu/citizens-initiative/public/welcome (accessed 12 December 2016).

European Commission. (2015b). Communication from the Commission on the European Citizens' Initiative 'Stop Vivisection'. http://ec.europa.eu/environment/chemicals/lab_animals/pdf/vivisection/en.pdf (accessed 12 December 2016).

European Commission. (2016). Attitudes of Europeans towards Animal Welfare. Special Eurobarameter 442. doi:10.2875/884639.

Gjerris, M. (2015). Willed blindness: A discussion of our moral shortcomings in relation to animals. *Jornal of Agricultural and Environmental Ethics*, 28: 517–532.

Graça, J., Calheiros, M. M. & Oliveira, A. (2014). Moral disengagement in harmful but cherished food practices? An exploration into the case of meat. *Journal of Agricultural and Environmental Ethics*, 27: 749–765.

Harrison, R. (1964). *Animal machines: The new factory farming industry*. London: Vincent Stuart Publishers.

Herzog, H., Rowan, A. N. & Kossow, D. (2001). Social attitudes and animals,. In D. J. Salem & A. N. Rowan (eds.), *The state of the animals* (pp. 55–69). Washington, DC: Humane Society Press.

Kleveland, L. (2005). Platforms and Funds for Alternatives to Animal Experimentation. A report from The Norwegian Reference Centre for Laboratory Animal Science & Alternatives, Norwegian School of Veterinary Science,

Oslo, Norway. http://oslovet.norecopa.no/platform/report/ecopaplatforms.pdf (accessed 12 December 2016).

Leaman, J., Latter, J. & Clemence, M. (2014). Attitudes to animal research in 2014. A report by Ipsos MORI for the Department for Business, Innovation & Skills, https://www.ipsos-mori.com/Assets/Docs/Polls/sri_BISanimalresearch_NONTRENDreport.pdf (accessed 12 December 2016).

Lund, T. B. (2011). Painful dilemmas. PhD thesis. Institute of Food and Resource Economics, University of Copenhagen. p.159.

Lund, T. B., Lassen, J. & Sandøe, P. (2012). Public attitude formation regarding animal research. *Anthrozoös*, 25: 475–490.

Lund, T. B., Mørkbak, M. R., Lassen, J. & Sandøe, P. (2014). Painful dilemmas: A study of the way the public's assessment of animal research balances costs to animals against human benefits. *Public Understanding of Science*, 23: 428–444.

Meijboom L. B. F. & Stassen E. N. (eds.). (2016). *The end of animal life: A start for ethical Debate. Ethical and societal considerations on killing animals.* Wageningen: Wageningen Academic Press.

National Centre for the Replacement Refinement & Reduction of Animals in Research (NC3RC). (2014). Annual report. London. http://nc3rs.org.uk/annualreport2014/.

National Centre for the Replacement Refinement & Reduction of Animals in Research (NC3RC). (2015). Responsibility in the use of animals in bioscience research: Expectations of the major research council and charitable funding bodies. https://www.mrc.ac.uk/publications/browse/responsibility-in-the-use-of-animals-in-research/ (accessed 12 December 2016).

Nielsen, A. P., Lassen, J. & Sandøe, P. (2004). Involving the public – participatory methods and democratic ideals. *Global Bioethics*, 17: 191–201.

Nielsen, A. P., Lassen, J. & Sandøe, P. (2007). Democracy at its best? The consensus conference in a cross-national perspective. *Journal of Agricultural and Environmental Ethics*, 20: 13–35.

Nielsen, A. P. & Sandøe, P. (2007). Democracy at its best? The consensus conference in a cross-national perspective. *Journal of Agricultural and Environmental Ethics*, 20: 13–35.

Röcklinsberg, H., Gamborg, C. & Gjerris, M. (2014). A case for integrity: Gains from including more than animal welfare in animal ethics committee deliberations. *Laboratory Animals*, 48: 61–71.

Röcklinsberg, H. (2015). Lay persons involvement and public interest. Ethical assessment in animal ethics committees in Sweden. The Swedish Transition Process of the EU Directive 2010/63/EU With Regard to Harm-Benefit Analysis in Animal Ethics Committees. *ALTEX Proceedings*, 4(1): 45–48.

Rollin, B. E. (2006). The regulation of animal research and the emergence of animal ethics: A conceptual history. *Theoretical Medicine and Bioethics*, 27: 285–304.

Rowe, G. & Frewer, L. J. (2000). Public participation methods: A framework for evaluation. *Science, Technology & Human Values*, 25: 3–29.

Sandøe, P. & Christiansen, S. B. (2008). *Ethics of animal use*. Oxford: Blackwell.

Schuppli, C. A. (2011). Decisions about the use of animals in research: Ethical reflection by animal ethics committee members. *Anthrozoös*, 24: 409–425.

Stop Vivisection (2015). http://www.stopvivisection.eu (accessed 12 December 2016).

van Asselt Marjolein, B. & Rijkens-Klomp, N. (2002). A look in the mirror: Reflection on participation in integrated assessment from a methodological perspective. *Global Environmental Change*, 12: 167–184.

Vapnek, J. & Chapman, M. (2010). *Legislative and regulatory options for animal welfare*. Rome: Food and Agriculture Organization for the United Nations.

Vieira de Castro, A. C. & Olsson, I. A. (2015). Does the goal justify the methods? Harm and benefit in neuroscience research using animals. *Current Topics in Behavioral Neurosciences*, 19: 47–78.

von Roten, F. C. (2009). European attitudes towards animal research overview and consequences for science. *Science Technology & Society*, 14: 349–364.

7 The Future of Animal Research: Guesstimates on Technical and Ethical Developments

With Jan Lund Ottesen

Most people will probably agree that a future world where we do not have to use animals in research will, all things being equal, be a better world to live in. But as long as one accepts that animal research to at least some extent is necessary to e.g. obtain basic knowledge for better understanding the human (and animal) physiology, to produce safe and better medicines for patients with severe diseases and to test necessary chemicals for toxicity, the prerequisite for such an ideal world is the development of the right alternatives to laboratory animals. With such alternatives at hand the use of animals for research purposes would not be necessary.

The present EU legislation covering the use of animals for experimental purposes (Directive 2010/63/EU) already lays down in Recital 10 that the ultimate goal is to replace all animals in experiments: The Directive represents an important step towards achieving the final goal of full replacement of procedures on live animals for scientific and educational purposes as soon as it is scientifically possible to do so (European Commission, 2010). Even though total replacement of experimental animals realistically is not within reach for the next decade(s), it is still possible to do better than today. In this chapter we look at the developing trends within the area of laboratory animal use and present the possible ethical discussions that these can give rise to.

7.1 NEW REFINEMENTS

The enclosures where we house laboratory animals today (cages, pens etc.) are where the animals in most cases spend the majority of their lives. It is therefore an obvious good place to begin to improve the lives of the animals we use. There is no global legislation dictating the minimum housing conditions, so in many places there is definitely room for improvement to ensure that the best possible housing conditions are provided to the animals. Within EU the tiny 'shoebox cages' to house mice that were allowed in the previous EU legislation are no longer accepted. It also seems likely that as the present legislation is developed further, the minimum cage sizes for mice and rats will continue to expand. There is no reason to believe that even those of today's facilities that have state-of-the-art conditions cannot be further improved. Similar to the fact that the state-of-the-art facilities we had 20 years ago were not as good as the ones we see today, the future housing of laboratory animals will probably also look better than today.

Optimal housing conditions represent one key element in the 'refinement' part of the 3Rs. Another equally important area is ensuring that the animals we use do not feel more pain than absolutely necessary. Every effort must be made to ensure that pain is minimized. For some animal models it is furthermore a dilemma that the inflammation that results in pain is part of the model and analgesic drugs, having anti-inflammatory qualities, cannot be supplied. But what if it were possible in the future to create genetically modified animals that could not feel the pain? This is not pure science fiction. Several different genetically modified mouse models have been created where the mice are still sensitive to pain, but have no perception of it (i.e. they do not avoid situations where they experience such pain) (Sun et al., 2009). So in theory it should be possible to create animals that do not feel pain. We return to the ethical discussion of creating such animals later in this chapter.

7.2 NEW REPLACEMENTS

In chapter six of their famous book, *The Principles of Humane Experimental Technique*, that introduced the 3R concept, Russel and Burch (1959, p. 105) wrote: 'Desirable as replacement is, it would be a mistake to put all our humanitarian eggs in this basket alone. The progress of replacement is gradual, nor is it ever likely to absorb the whole of experimental biology.' The development since then has proven them right. There has been a gradual replacement of animals with non-animal models, although some think this process is moving too slow given current technological advances. With the growing public attention to animal welfare and the growing costs of using laboratory animals, it seems reasonable to imagine that the future will bring a continued and even accelerated development where non-animal models will replace at least some if not all laboratory animals.

In most cases the use of a validated cell culture is a much less expensive way of testing than using animals is (not taking the expenses to develop and validate the cell culture model into the equation) and normally also with much less variation in the results. Furthermore, much less of the compound in question is normally needed for in vitro tests, which is another argument to prefer such vitro assays. To understand the slow progress in the area, it is necessary to understand that the key word here is *validation*. Today there are simply not enough validated cell culture models to get the answers you can obtain when using animals. The future will probably see more of such validated non-animal models, but as many of the animal models are used to ensure human safety, there has been a regulative hesitation, as societies have not been willing to take any chances. It has to be almost more than certain (validated) that the in vitro assays produce results that are as reliable as the data obtained using animals. However, if it is believed that a cell culture will be able to result in just as reliable an answer as an animal model is, then there is both an economical and a scientific benefit to use such assays.

Some of these assays are already used extensively today (e.g. in the pharmaceutical industry) to test the thousands of new compounds being produced in laboratories around the globe. Many of these compounds are initially screened in non-animal models such as receptor binding assays or cell proliferation assays, and only the relatively few compounds that have the right properties in the in vitro assays are further evaluated in animals. If these non-animal assays were not available, undoubtedly more animals would be used to test compounds than is the case today, as some of these compounds later would fail as candidates for new drugs because they did not result in receptor binding or had uncontrolled cell proliferation and therefore could not be used in patients. The pharmaceutical industry is thus already using non-animal assays to a large extent, but these assays do not replace any animals in the yearly 'statistics' because no animals are used for this initial screening of potential candidates anyway.

Cell assays containing only one cell type will obviously only result in information from that particular cell type, and it is often claimed that you do not get the same complex interplay between different organ systems in such cell assays as you get in a laboratory animal. In the future it could, however, be possible to have combinations of different in vitro assays giving more 'complex answers'. Huge efforts are presently put into developing a 'human on a chip'. Initially most of the research is directed into developing different models: organs on a chip like 'lung on a chip', 'heart on a chip', kidney on a chip' etc. where a micro device – no bigger than a computer memory stick or a microscope slide – will have the human cells you want to utilize (lung, heart, kidney, etc.) combined with e.g. blood- or air flow so they mimic the mechanical, chemical and physiological functions of the similar human cells in the specific organs of the body. By combining some of these 'organs on a chip' you could begin to have a 'human on a chip'. A lot of research and validation is still needed before this will replace a significant number of animals, but that these technologies in the future will replace animals seems likely as long as the necessary resources are invested to develop them (Hansjorg Wyss Institute, 2015).

7.3 IN SILICO (COMPUTER) MODELS REPLACING ANIMAL STUDIES

Mathematical calculations and computer-based analysis are already being used to predict whether new compounds or medical substances produced in laboratories have the looked-for properties, and they are used for risk assessments. Such mathematical models (biosimulations) can give insights into how quickly a compound/medicine is taken up into the blood stream or how long it takes to diffuse into tissue. One of the more promising areas is the quantitative structure-activity relationship (QSAR) modelling that uses mathematical modelling on a large number of previous data to get statistical relationship between toxicity (or pharmacological effect) of a chemical (or pharmaceutical) and its physiochemical (or pharmacological) properties and structural characteristics (Cherkasov *et al.*, 2014). With more and more data being captured and knowledge being gathered from these models combined with the history of computer power development that has so far followed what is called Moore's law (overall processing power for computers will double every two years), it seems likely that in the future even more precise predictions can be made using computers – thereby replacing animal models with computer models.

7.4 USE OF MANNEQUINS FOR EDUCATIONAL STUDIES

The future will probably bring more use of non-animal models for educational purposes. This is a practice that has been known for a long time: medical and veterinary students have always practised surgical knots on a 'dishcloth' before trying for the first time on laboratory animals – and patients! However, due to – among other factors – pressure from animal welfare and animal rights groups to completely abolish use of animals for educational purposes, models have been developed that in some cases can be used to reflect the real-life situation and be used as practice tools (Figure 7.1). There is no reason to expect that the technical development in this field should not continue and produce even better models than are available today.

Interactive computer animations can also work as models e.g. for demonstrating how the anatomy of the animals looks before the actual surgery is being performed. For some educations it is necessary to use models – especially for students in elementary school or high school, where the students are taught general subjects and most of them do not know what kind of education they will end up taking – as Directive 2010/63/EU, Article 5 limits animal use in education to higher education or training for vocational skills. For some educational experiments it can be argued that there is no extra gain in seeing/performing a real-life experiment compared to watching it on a computer (e.g. some of the classical physiology studies using frogs to measure contractile muscle responses resulting from an applied electrical stimulus). There are differing opinions on the degree to which animals can be replaced in e.g. the training of veterinarians and medical doctors, but most agree that it is possible to some extent. A study among veterinary students thus showed that if the students began by performing surgery on teddy bears, they became more self-assured when performing surgery on real animals – thus reducing unnecessary suffering (Langebæk *et al.*, 2012).

7.5 WILL THE TOTAL NUMBER OF ANIMALS IN RESEARCH DECREASE OR INCREASE IN THE FUTURE?

As mentioned at the beginning of this chapter, the European Union has as the ultimate goal the replacement of all animals used for experimental purposes, and many resources are being invested into this. From this perspective one can reasonably expect a decrease in the numbers of animals used in the future. However, before this is reached (not to speak of the total replacement of animals), the total number of animals used could instead increase to begin with. Critics could initially argue that this is a failure and that there needs to be more focus on replacing animals with non-sentient beings/mannequins, cell cultures etc. and reducing the number of animals. It should, however, be noted that both situations can actually exist at the same time. Russell and Burch did not talk about a reduction in total numbers when they put the 3R principles forward more than 50 years ago. They wrote: 'Reduction means reduction in the numbers of animals used to obtain information of a given amount and precision' (Russell and Burch, 1959, p. 64) (i.e. use of fewer animals than previously in a similar experimental setup while getting similar or better scientific quality of results). An increase in the total number of animals used can reflect that more or better research results are obtained. And especially with

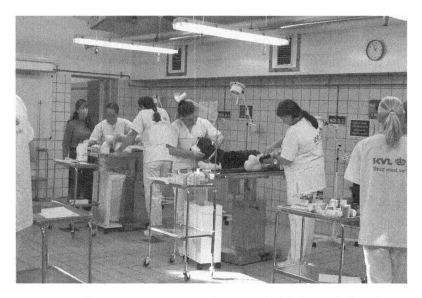

FIGURE 7.1 Reflection on new ways to replace animals, refining methods and avoiding unnecessary suffering is a continuous challenge.

Source: Photo: Rikke Langebæk.

the development of biotechnological tools such as genetic modification and cloning, it is now possible to perform research that was not possible previously, driving the total number of animals used upwards at the same time that it may be reduced within the individual projects.

With the initiatives mentioned in this chapter – and future initiatives that cannot be envisioned today – the ideal world that was introduced at the beginning of this chapter, where the use of any laboratory animals becomes unnecessary, seems less unrealistic than one would perhaps think, even though it admittedly lies many years into the future. But already now many interesting opportunities to replace animals with non-animal models can be seen – and a use of animals that takes greater care of their welfare and has greater respect for their nature can be envisioned.

7.6 ETHICAL DISCUSSIONS REGARDING USE OF LABORATORY ANIMALS IN THE FUTURE

The use of animals in research has from the beginning been seen as ethical controversial by those who believe that animals are ethical beings in their own right. With the growing focus on animal welfare and animal rights in Western societies, it is relatively safe to foresee that ethical discussions on the use of research animals will continue until the last laboratory animal is used.

From a utilitarian perspective, the growing understanding of the complexity of animal behaviour and needs will continue to challenge researchers to develop alternatives to animal experimentation. The more we grasp the complexity of animal sentience, the harder it becomes from this perspective to justify subjecting the animals to harmful experiments. Demands for better housing and pain management will probably continue to rise as well, driven by public demand and politicians trying to cater to it. From a utilitarian perspective, such higher standards required for the use of animals have to be balanced against what can be gained from using the animals. The goal is to maximize welfare overall, and the increasing opportunities that the development within biotechnologies such as genetic modification and cloning give researchers an opportunity to design animals as disease models for research purposes that have not been possible before. The utilitarian evaluation will thus have both to take into consideration the assumed welfare loss for the animals and the assumed gains for humans.

Animal rights groups with the ethical prima facie rule that humans have no right to use animals to further their own interests will continue to oppose all use of research animals. This pressure will probably also lead to increased demands for convincingly arguing the value of the intended research to animal ethical committees, higher demands for demonstrating real intent to implement the 3Rs and higher demands for adhering to ethical standards from funding agencies and journals when publishing the results. As the number of alternatives increase and their quality improve, animal rights groups will gain momentum in a debate climate where the need to justify is increasingly on the ones that wish to use animals – and researchers will increasingly have to argue the necessity of research to maintain broad public support.

These developments will challenge current research practices in more basic and explorative research fields in which researchers have no well-defined practical goals with the research, and it could be increasingly hard to find support for this kind of research as demands for the usefulness of the 'sacrifice' of the animals will grow – even though from a research perspective this kind of basic research is often a prerequisite for doing applied research with well-defined goals. Along the same line it is likely that researchers will have to be more careful when making claims about possible outcomes, as failure to reach intended goals will be less acceptable. Both developments might decrease opportunities to do research and might in and of themselves drive forward the development of alternatives to animals.

As mentioned earlier, the socio-zoological scale plays a large role when it comes to how the use of research animals is viewed. The lower on the scale an animal is placed by the majority in a society, the more the research becomes acceptable. The use of animals such as dogs, cats and non-human primates will thus be increasingly controversial, as the intimate relations between such animals and humans will be seen as more or less prohibitive for using them in research. Regarding the use of rodents and fish, one can also envision a growing concern as knowledge of the complexity of the sentience of these animals becomes more widespread.

These developments do, however, need to be balanced up against the increased role that research animals can play in diagnostics, alleviation of human pain and suffering and treatment of human diseases through biotechnologies such as genetic modification and cloning, not to mention research that is directed at animal health (e.g. developing vaccines for production animals). The utilitarian weighing of animal vs. human interests (or animal vs. animal interests) will thus continue, but the possible suffering created and the possible results gained may be even harder to estimate than today. To this can be added that many citizens within the EU find biotechnologies to be ethically problematic in themselves, although less so within research and medicine than within food production.

It was mentioned earlier that it might be possible to use the technologies to create e.g. mice that would not have the ability to experience pain. From a strictly utilitarian perspective, such an animal would be ideal, as the animal could be used for certain types of experiments without suffering negative welfare as a consequence of it. However, it is not hard to imagine the ethical discussions that could grow out of such an attempt to create an animal that would be deprived of one of the most important abilities of an animal seen from an evolutionary perspective. Undoubtedly some would find this a grotesque albeit logical way to end animal suffering in relation to research and oppose it from a range of ethical perspectives.

Using animals in research will continue to be an ethical challenge, and there is little doubt that the demands from society towards the research world in relation to a responsible use of animals will grow. At the same time, however, demands for better diagnostics, medicine and therapies will also continue to grow, and it will be the task of researchers, politicians, stakeholders and the citizens in general to take the time to discuss the ethical aspects of this development and strike a balance in legislation and practice that will be seen as socially robust. Otherwise the research communities accustomed to using animals might suddenly find that this way of gaining knowledge will be fundamentally challenged by societies in which the welfare and rights of animals play an increasing role.

QUESTIONS FOR DISCUSSION AND REFLECTION

1. Have you during education and training discussed, been introduced to or trained to use alternatives to animals?
2. What are the most important barriers to use and develop alternatives to animals within your area of research? Are they of practical or ethical kind?
3. What do you think will be the main ethical issues related to the use of animals in research in the near future?

REFERENCES

Cherkasov, A., Muratov, E. N., Fourches, D., Varnek, A., Baskin, I. I., Cronin, M., Dearden, J., Gramatica, P., Martin, Y. C. & Todeschini, R. (2014). QSAR modeling: Where have you been? Where are you going to? *Journal of Medicinal Chemistry*, 57: 4977–5010.

European Commission. (2010). Directive 2010/63/EU on the protection of animals used for scientific purposes. Official Journal of the European Union. L276: 33–79. http://eur-lex.europa.eu/LexUriServ/LexUriServ.do?uri=OJ:L:2010:276:00 33:0079:en:pdf (accessed 12 December 2016).

Hansjorg Wyss Institute. (2015). Lung-on-a-chip. Harvard University.

Langebæk, R., Eika, B., Jensen, A. L., Tanggaard, L., Toft, N. & Berendt, M. (2012). Anxiety in veterinary surgical students: A quantitative study. *Journal of Veterinary Medical Education*, 39: 331–340.

Russell, W. & Burch, R. (1959). *The principles of humane experimental technique.* London: Methuen & Co. Ltd.

Sun, Y.-G., Gracias, N. G., Drobish, J. K., Vasko, M. R., Gereau, R. W. & Chen, Z.-F. (2009). The c-kit signaling pathway is involved in the development of persistent pain. *PAIN*, 144: 178–186.

Index

Printed in the United States
by Baker & Taylor Publisher Services